Advances in Clinical Neuropsychology

Volume 2

Advances in Clinical Neuropsychology

Volume 2

Edited by

Ralph E. Tarter

University of Pittsburgh School of Medicine
Western Psychiatric Institute and Clinic
Pittsburgh, Pennsylvania

and

Gerald Goldstein

Veterans Administration Highland Drive Medical Center and
University of Pittsburgh School of Medicine
Western Psychiatric Institute and Clinic
Pittsburgh, Pennsylvania

Plenum Press • New York and London

ISBN 0-306-41722-7

©1984 Plenum Press, New York
A Division of Plenum Publishing Corporation
233 Spring Street, New York, N.Y. 10013

Printed in the United States of America

PREFACE

This second volume of the series **Advances in Clinical Neuro-psychology** addresses the neurological and neuropsychological disorders that are seen most frequently in children. The book begins with a discussion of normal and abnormal brain development. From there, neurological and neuropsychological assessment methods are described and evaluated. The main body of the text is concerned with reviewing the major childhood disorders, and includes discussions of brain trauma, dyslexia, minimal brain dysfunction, mental retardation and epilepsy. These latter conditions adversely impact on psychosocial development and limit educational attainment. Approaching these disorders from a neurobehavioral perspective, therefore, potentially has ramifications for improving detection and assessment procedures, as well as for developing new intervention strategies.

This book continues the tradition of the first volume in that the contents include topics that address basic research, as well as clinical problems. It is hoped that this combination will encourage the professional to integrate research and clinical application in guiding their investigative activities or clinical endeavors.

A number of individuals have facilitated the efforts of the editors in producing this ongoing series, and have particularly contributed to this volume. Our appreciation is expressed to Dr. Thomas Detre and to the Office of Education and Regional Programming at Western Psychiatric Institute and Clinic. In this regard, the help of Dr. Jeannette Jerrell in organizing the conference, upon which this book is partially based, is acknowledged. Gratitude is expressed to Cheryl Schmitt, Administrative Specialist at Western Psychiatric Institute and Clinic for her enthusiastic support, and to her staff for preparing the manuscript. The collective effort of Theresa Cukanow, Karen Alexander, Cyndi Meister, Margaret Malloy, Michele Bevilacqua, Debbie Reichbaum, and Marty Levine is sincerely acknowledged. The secretarial assistance provided by Lorraine Hummel of the Veterans Administration Hospital is also appreciated. However, it was the inexorable editorial, text compositing, and administrative effort expended by Kathy Lou Edwards which was responsible for transforming this project from a plan to a product. The support of the Veterans Administration throughout this project to Dr. Goldstein is also earnestly acknowledged. Finally, the editors express their deepest appreciation to the chapter authors for their contributions, and for their interest in and support of this project.

January 1984
Ralph E. Tarter, Ph.D.
Gerald Goldstein, Ph.D.

Pittsburgh, Pennsylvania

CONTENTS

NORMAL AND ABNORMAL DEVELOPMENT OF THE BRAIN

Roger Williams and Verne S. Caviness, Jr.

Harvard Medical School
Southard Laboratory, Eunice Kennedy Shriver Center
Harvard Medical School
Waltham, Massachusetts

The gestational period is exceptionally hazardous, having a particularly high mortality rate during the first trimester. Morbidity is also high, with an incidence of developmental abnormalities approaching five percent of all live births (Niswander & Gordon, 1972). The central nervous system is especially vulnerable (Leck, Record, McKeown, & Edwards, 1968; Creasy & Alberman, 1976). The severity of the public health problem posed by developmental disorders of the nervous system is underscored by the fact that in the United States alone over three percent or approximately six million individuals are affected (Moser & Wolf, 1971).

This chapter will briefly review the salient milestones of normal brain development, and provide some illustrative examples of developmental disorders thought to arise during the epoch. Emphasis will be placed upon the cerebral cortex. This stems from the general assumption that abnormalities of behavior, learning, affect, language and perception, as well as the epilepsies, reflect at some level abnormalities of the function and, probably, the structure of the cerebral cortex.

NORMAL STRUCTURE OF THE CEREBRAL CORTEX

A few introductory remarks about the normal structure of the cerebral cortex are in order. The elemental structural and functional unit is the neuron. The cortex consists of billions of neurons distributed to a depth of two to six millimeters over the entire cerebral surface. Cortical neurons are classified into a finite number of subspecies based upon similarities in size and overall shape. Neuronal classifications depend in large measure on the histological method employed. The most popular utilized

1

analine dyes (e.g., cresyl violet, hematoxylin-eosin) that stain
nucleic acids confined largely to the nucleus and adjacent cyto-
plasm. These methods disclose three general cell types and are
illustrated in Figure 1. First, there are neurons which are tri-
angular or "pyramidal" in shape. Second, there are neurons which
are smaller and more round or "granular" in surface contour. And
third, there are neurons which are more variable or
"polymorphic." Although these analine dyes have been very useful
for delineating cellular organization and histological reaction,
they provide a very incomplete view of neuronal structure, revealing no more than five percent of the surface area of cortical neurons.

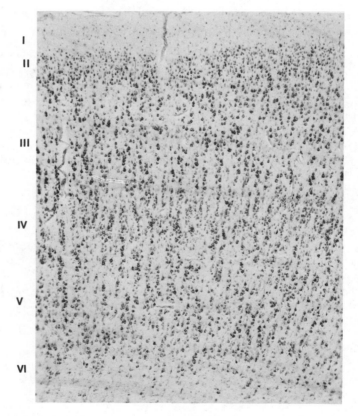

Fig. 1. Photomicrograph illustrating the typical six layers of
          typical neocortex from the parietal lobe of a four year
          old child stained by the cresyl violet (CV) method.
          (64X).

The cytologic method developed by Golgi over one hundred years ago provides the optimum means for examining the entire surface area of individual neurons (Lorente de No, 1949). The rapid Golgi method depends upon the intracytoplasmic precipitation of silver chromate salts which fill the cell body and cytoplasmic envelope of axonal and dendritic processes. (As viewed in Golgi preparations, individual cortical neurons have a more complex external morphology and are illustrated in Figure 2.) A stout dendrite emerges from the apex of pyramidal neurons and ascends through the suprajacent layers to ramify under the pial surface. Each apical dendrite gives off a number of subordinate oblique branches, and an elaborate dendritic arbor emerges also from the base of each pyramid. The dendritic processes of the pyramidal neurons are studded with small spiny processes. An axon emerges from the base of the pyramidal cell, and after giving off a number of collateral branches, exits into the subcortical white matter. Granular non-pyramidal neurons have multiple somatic dendrites oriented into a variety of shapes (Jones, 1975), and short axons with abundant collaterals which participate in local intracortical circuits. The dendrites of non-pyramidal local circuit neurons are largely non-spiny. Polymorphic neurons share in varying degree the dendrite and axonal morphological features of pyramidal and non-pyramidal neurons.

Companion electron microscopic studies of cortical neurons disclose that axons terminate upon the dendrites and cell bodies of other neurons by specialized synaptic contacts. Synapses are classified into a variety of morphological subtypes based upon the shape of their neurotransmitter containing vesicles and the symmetry of their pre- and postsynaptic membrane thickenings (Colonnier, 1981). Where morphological subtype has been correlated with function, synapses classified as "asymmetric" are excitatory, and "symmetric" are inhibitory in function. Asymmetrical, presumably excitatory synapses, are most numerous on pyramidal cell dendritic spines, and may number in the tens of thousands for each cell. Symmetrical, presumably inhibitory synapses, are fewer in number and are concentrated on the smooth surfaces of proximal dendrites, the cell body and the initial portion of the axon. Symmetrical and asymmetrical synaptic terminals are distributed more evenly along the smooth dendritic surfaces of local circuit neurons.

When viewed in histological sections oriented orthogonally to the surface, the cerebral cortex is seen to be composed of two or more concentric layers formed of cells and their fibrous processes (Nauta & Karten, 1970). It is a remarkable architectural feature of neocortex that the component neurons are ordered according to their cell class into five successive parallel planes or laminae. These are demonstrated in Figures 1 and 3. They lie below an outer "molecular" or "plexiform" layer which contains axons and

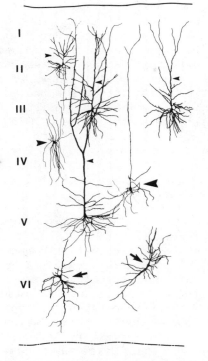

Fig. 2.   Camera lucida drawings of representative Golgi impreg-
           nated neurons from human neocortex. The apical shifts
           (small arrowheads) of pyramidal neurons in layers II-V
           ascend to ramify in layer I. Stellate local circuit
           neurons (large arrowheads) are pictured here in layers
           III and IV, and polymorphic non-pyramidal neurons
           (triple arrowheads) are in layer VI.

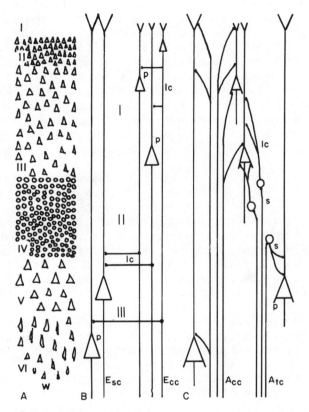

Fig. 3.   Schematic representation of cell pattern (A) and the
           organization of connections (B,C) of normal neocortex.
           The roman numerals at left in A identify the six neo-
           cortical laminae. The roman numerals in B represent
           the three cellular tiers. Pyramidal cells (p) of the
           upper tier are the principal targets, as well as the
           principal cells of origin of cortico-cortical afferent
           (Acc) and efferent (Ecc) axonal systems, respectively.
           Pyramidal neurons of the lower tier are the cells of
           origin of subcortical efferent systems (Esc). Stellate
           neurons (s) in C are the principal targets of thalamo-
           cortical afferents (Atc). Local cortical circuits (lc)
           are formed by collaterals of axons of the pyramidal neu-
           rons in tier I. These contact other pyramidal neurons
           of the same tier, as well as those of the lower tier.
           Another major local circuit is formed by the axons of
           stellate cell(s) which form connections with pyramidal
           neurons of the upper and lower tiers.

dendrites, but few nerve cell bodies. Neocortical layers II and III are formed by small to medium-sized pyramidal neurons, respectively, which give rise to the majority of connections between cortical regions within the same and between the two cerebral hemispheres (Jones, 1981). Granular local circuit neurons are found throughout the cellular layer, but in many areas are concentrated heavily at mid-cortical levels into a distinct layer IV. In most regions of the neocortex, layer V contains larger pyramidal cells which give rise to all projections of the neocortex which descend below the thalamus to brainstem and spinal cord. Many of the polymorphic neurons which are concentrated in layer VI are the origin of axonal connections between neocortex and thalamus.

There are local differences in this general laminar pattern which are distributed continuously across the cerebral surface, and are topologically similar among members of the same species. Regional variations in cortical cell and fiber pattern have been used by anatomists for almost a century to parcellate the cortex into a variety of subordinate areas (Brazier & Petsche, 1978). These anatomically distinctive cortical sectors have different patterns of synaptic connections and probably subserve different functions (Caviness & Frost, 1981).

Although the laminar arrangement of neurons in the tangential plane has traditionally received the greatest emphasis, there is also a significant columnar organization in the cortical dimension (Von Bonin & Mehler, 1971). The orientation of individual neurons into discrete radial columns is most explicit in the immature cortex and becomes less distinct as growth and differentiation progress. Figures 1,4 and 5 illustrate this process. In the same cortical sub-field, neurons of similar size and shape are in tangential register on adjacent columns, accounting for the characteristic laminar pattern. Each anatomical column is narrow, usually no more than a few cells in diameter. These "micro" columns are probably the building blocks for the functional columnar units which have been defined neurophysiologically (Mountcastle, 1979).

NORMAL DEVELOPMENT OF THE CEREBRAL CORTEX

Development of the mammalian cerebral cortex is a remarkable feat of biological engineering. Many of the salient steps were predicted by histologists of the last century, such as Kolliker (1896) and Cajal (1911). Technological advances in neuroscience over the last twenty years have, for the first time, provided the methods for testing these hypotheses and have generated many new ones. Details of this exciting chapter in developmental neurobiology are reviewed elsewhere (Sidman & Rakic, 1973; Lemire, Loeser, Leech, & Alvord, 1975; Jacobson, 1978; Rakic, 1981; Volpe, 1981). Only the highlights will be mentioned here.

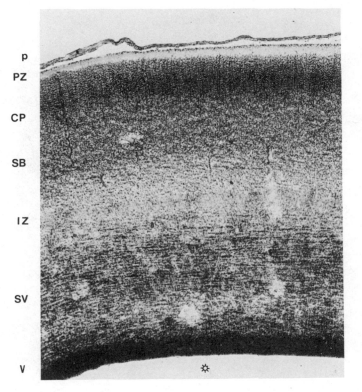

Fig. 4.   Photomicrograph through the developing cerebral wall of
           a 14 week human fetus. The asterisk marks the ventricu-
           lar cavity, V and SV are the ventricular and sub-ven-
           tricular germinal zones, respectively. IZ is the inter-
           mediate zone containing migrating neurons, glial and
           neuronal processes. SB is the subplate, CP the cortical
           plate and PZ is the plexiform or molecular layer. An
           arrow points to the developing pia and arachnoid mem-
           branes. (H&E, 100X).

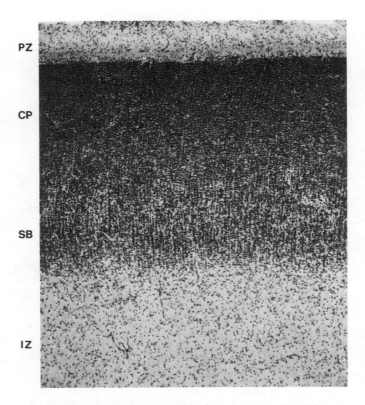

Fig. 5.   Low power photomicrograph through frontal neocortex of a
human fetus at 20 weeks gestation. The normal radially
striate appearance due to cellular "micro-columns" is
evident, but the typical six laminae are not yet developed. Cells in the subplate (SB) and depths of the
cortical plate (CP) have commenced growth and differentiation, and hence are further apart than the less
mature neurons of the superficial CP. (H&E, 150X).

Neurogenesis and histogenesis. Neurogenesis refers to the formation of nerve cells, while histogenesis refers to the events through which cells are assembled into the individual tissue components of the nervous system. In the majority of regions of the human fetal nervous system, including the cerebral neocortex, these events are compressed into the first half of pregnancy (Sidman & Rakic, 1973; Dobbing & Sands, 1973). It is essential to keep in mind that these early dramatic events in the formation of the cerebral cortex are paralleled by equally critical events in the formation of supporting tissues. The blood vascular system, the choroid plexus at the margins of the ventricles, the mesenchymal membranes around the nervous system and the skull are also formed during this period. Normal development of the cerebral hemispheres is dependent upon adequate vascular perfusion and the normal formation and circulation of cerebrospinal fluid. In addition to their nutritive and waste disposal functions these two circulatory systems probably provide a balance of hydraulic forces necessary for proper support and molding of the developing nervous system (Desmond & Jacobson, 1977).

The primordial neuroectoderm differentiates in the third gestational week and evolves into a tubular structure lined by proliferating cells. Closure of the anterior and posterior poles of the neural tube is accomplished by the end of the fourth week, and the brain develops from the anterior pole. At least at these early developmental stages, normal brain development is critically dependent upon normal interaction with differentiating tissues of the face and nasopharynx (Jacobson, 1978).

The development of the cerebral cortex commences at six to seven weeks gestation after the evagination of the telencephalic vesicles. All neurons and glial supporting cells arise from the proliferative neuroepithelium lining the ventricular cavities. Virtually the entire population of cortical neurons in the adult human brain are generated before twenty weeks gestation. As they become postmitotic, young neurons are simple bipolar forms which appear to be freely motile. This is illustrated in Figure 6. They must reach their final destination at the cortical surface by migrating over a terrain which increases in size and complexity as development progresses. The most compelling hypothesis as to how this difficult task is accomplished has been reviewed by Rakic (1981).

One of the first cells to differentiate in the developing cerebrum has the morphological and antigenic characteristics of a specialized glial cell. Note in Figure 7 that its cell body lies just above the ventricular germinal zone, and has inwardly and outwardly directed cytoplasmic processes. The inward process attaches to cells lining the ventricular surface, and the longer process directed radially outward attaches to blood vessels and

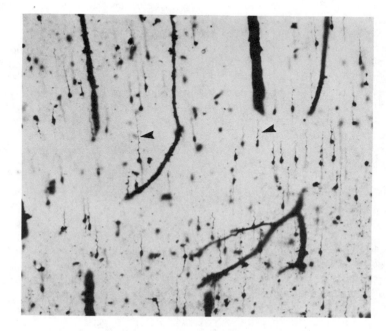

Fig. 6.   Photomicrograph through the intermediate zone of an 18-
           week human fetus impregnated by the Golgi method. The
           branched tubular structures are impregnated blood ves-
           sels, and multiple bipolar young neurons can be seen
           migrating through the field. Without exception, migrat-
           ing neurons are oriented radially outward with their
           slender leading processes (arrowheads) addressing the
           cortical surface which is above the field of view. In
           contrast to Figure 7, in this section the impregnation
           favored migrating neurons and radial glial processes did
           not impregnate. (Golgi-Cos, 250X).

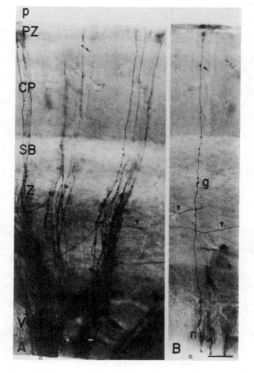

Fig. 7.   Photomicrographs through the developing cerebral wall of
a mouse fetus illustrating the spoke-like configuration
of the processes of radial glial cells. In A, several
radial glial processes are impregnated and wander in and
out of focus as they extend upward to terminate at the
pial surface (p). In B, a single fiber is favorably
illustrated and its cell body (n), which is slightly out
of focus, is seen to reside in the ventricular zone.
The radial glial processes are unbranched until they terminate at the pial surface, but give rise to a number of
lamellate processes (arrows). Impregnated developing
axons course across the field horizontally (arrowheads)
but no neurons are impregnated in the sections illustrated here.

mesenchymal cells at the cerebral surface. These specialized astrocytes, called "radial glia" by Rakic (1981), persist throughout
the developmental period, spanning the entire thickness of the
cerebral wall like the spokes of a wheel.

As viewed in the cytological preparations of Golgi, mentioned
above, the postmitotic young neurons are also oriented with stout
leading processes directed radially outward, and thin trailing
processes inward toward the ventricular surface (see Figure 6). In
favorable sections, young bipolar neurons are closely adjacent to
the processes of radial glial cells. When examined in serial
electron micrographs, the cytoplasmic membrane of migrating neurons is apposed to and partially envelops the radial glial processes, but not the processes of other neurons. Hence, migrating
young neurons seem to use radial glial fibers as guide wires in
their ascent to the cerebral surface. This process is illustrated
in Figure 8. This relationship implies a rather unique form of
cell-cell interaction, the details of which are still largely unknown and under vigorous investigation (PintoLord & Caviness,
1979).

Autoradiographic studies in laboratory animals confirm that
there is a systematic relationship between the date of birth and
laminar position of cortical neurons. Tritiated thymadine is administered to pregnant animals and is incorporated into the nuclei
of fetal cells. Those which are undergoing their last mitoses
during the time of pulse injection are labeled most heavily
(Rakic, 1981). When histological sections of the cerebral cortex
examined later are coated with a photographic emulsion, isotope
labeled nuclei activate the overlying silver grains. These studies disclose that the oldest cells occupy layer I and the inner-
most layer of the developing cortex. Neurons generated later occupy successively more superficial levels in the intervening
zone. This inside-out pattern of cortical formation implies that
cells which complete migration first must give up their glial attachments, allowing later migrating cells to pass by (see Figure
8). The discrete laminar pattern of labeled nuclei is preserved
at later stages of development, confirming that there is very
little shift in cellular position during growth and differentiation (Caviness, 1982).

When the developing cerebral cortex is examined at early
stages in Golgi impregnations, as illustrated in Figure 9, many of
the oldest neurons in the outer and inner-most layers already have
well differentiated dendrites and axons (Marin-Padilla, 1978).
These neurons ultimately reside in layers I, VI and perhaps V of
the more mature cortex. The number persisting in layer I decreases progressively around the time of birth and thereafter.

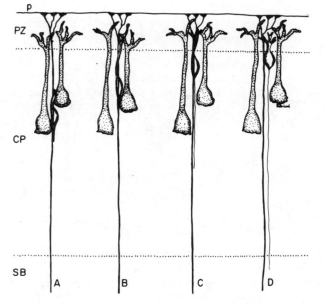

Fig. 8.   Schematic representation of the terminal phases of mi-
           gration (A–D) of a young neuron (darkly shaded) in the
           normal cortex. Post-migratory neurons (stippled) have
           minimal contact with the radial glial fiber and are
           readily displaced from its surface by the leading proc-
           ess of the migrating cell. After the leading process
           enters the plexiform zone (PZ) and begins to branch, the
           young neuron also becomes largely disengaged from the
           radial glial fiber. At or near the termination of mi-
           gration an axon is observed to descend from the inferior
           pole of the cell.

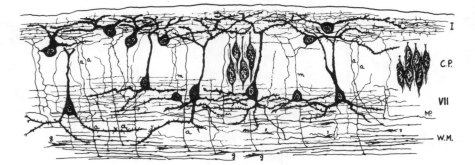

Fig. 9.   Composite camera lucida drawings of Golgi impregnated
           neurons from the immature neocortex of the fetal cat.
           Neurons of the plexiform zone (here labeled I) and sub-
           plate (here labeled VII) have well developed dendritic
           arbors and axons, and some have assumed a pyramidal
           shape. These are the earliest cells generated. By con-
           trast, neurons of the cortical plate (CP) retain their
           immature bipolar form. (From Marin-Padilla, 1978, with
           permission).

The developmental history of neurons destined for the intervening layers is different. Many of the earliest formed appear to
differentiate an axon from their inferior pole before they enter
the cortex proper (Shoukimas & Hinds, 1978), perhaps in response
to cues residing in the fibrous intermediate zone through which
they migrate. Differentiation of the leading process, by contrast,
commences only after it is delivered fully into the plexiform
molecular layer. As neurons become postmigratory and relinquish
their attachments to the glial guides, they are essentially
tethered in position by the differentiation of their leading process above and axon below (Pinto-Lord & Caviness, 1979). This
progression is revealed in Figure 10. Although the apical process
and axon continue to elongate, there is, until much later, little
or no further differentiation.

At this stage, the primordial cortex has three cardinal
layers (see Figures 5 and 9). The outer plexiform layer contains
abundant axonal fibers, many of which seem to be of brainstem origin, and a few differentiated neurons; the "cortical plate" contains tightly packed, radially oriented, relatively undifferenti-
ated postmigratory neurons; and, an inner zone or "subplate" which
is composed of differentiated neurons, fibers and migrating young
neurons. The cortical plate continues to grow by the addition of
new neurons until eighteen to twenty weeks gestation, at which
time neuronal proliferation and migration are virtually complete.

The migratory mechanism is a remarkable evolutionary device
which insures that many aspects of cortical development proceed
normally and efficiently. In addition to insuring that migrating
neurons get from one place to another, the radial glial guide
functions as a rigid two-point coordinate system. Hence, neurons
from genetically distinctive loci of the germinal epithelium arrive at topologically identical loci on the cortical surface. In
this way, genetic heterogeneity in the germinal epithelium is map-
ped faithfully on the cortex in the tangential plane. The inside-
out sequence of intracortical neuronal migration insures that temporal differences in gene expression are also preserved, but in
the radial dimension. The faithful transcription of spatially
distributed and temporally expressed genetic differences onto the
cortical surface may account, at least in part, for regional differences in cell and fiber architecture described above. Differentiation of the axon from the inferior pole of the cell during
migration, and of the apical pole of the cell at the end of migration, provides a mechanism for fixing cellular and fiber relationships throughout subsequent periods of growth and differentiation. The chain of events set in motion by guided migration provides the anatomical substrate which insures the functional integrity of individual columnar units and of the cerebrum as a whole.

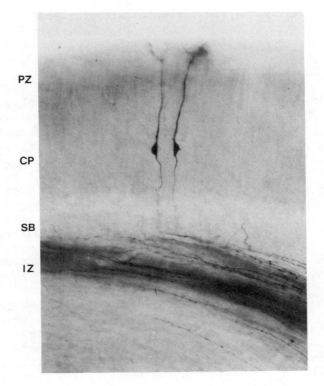

PZ

CP

SB

IZ

Fig. 10. Photomicrograph of two Golgi impregnated neurons in the
          cortical plate of the mouse embryo. They are tethered
          in place by differentiation of their leading processes
          in the plexiform zone and their axon which exists into
          the subcortical fiber plexus. (IZ) (Rapid Golgi, 250X).

Between ten and thirteen weeks gestation, the axons of some cortical neurons, many of which may still be migrating, grow toward the midline in discrete fiber bundles (Rakic & Yakovlev, 1968). They target upon a histologically unique zone just above the anterior wall of the third ventricle, where they are encouraged to cross the midline, and in this manner the major commissural systems of the forebrain develop. This is illustrated in Figure 11. The anterior commissure, connecting olfactory and medial temporal cortical structures, is the first to develop, followed by the hippocampal commissure. The remainder of the cortex is connected by the corpus callosum which has a more protracted developmental history. Recent studies in animals have shown that the distribution of callosal afferents in the cortex is initially diffuse, but is ultimately restricted so that cortical areas with the same cytoarchitecture and presumably the same function are connected reciprocally (Innocenti, Fiore, & Caminiti, 1977).

Neuronal Growth and Differentiation

Once committed to their definitive positions, and having achieved proper orientation, neurons enter a period of growth (Marin-Padilla, 1970). During this second epoch, their axonal and dendritic surfaces become linked together to form a stable pattern of innerconnections which are the basis of functional neuronal circuits. Far more young neurons are probably generated than will eventually inhabit the adult nervous system (Jacobson, 1978). Cells which are not recruited into stable connections die and are eliminated. In the human brain, the second epoch has an extended period which continues through the second half of pregnancy until maturity. Cells increase greatly in size and come to assume their characteristic adult shapes. Multiple glial cell species proliferate. Astrocytes differentiate and acquire the ability to elaborate fibrous processes in response to injury. The oligodendroglial cells elaborate the myelin sheath essential to the function of multiple axonal systems. The blood vascular system and cerebrospinal pathways achieve their definite configuration and physiologic characteristics. Maturation of the investing mesenchymal structures is marked, finally, by closure of the bony sutures of the skull.

Afferent fibers from thalamic relay nuclei grow outward toward the cortex early in development, and then seem to assume a "holding" pattern beneath the cortical plate for a period of many weeks (Rakic, 1977). Prior to sixteen to eighteen weeks gestation, the only synapses identifiable in the cortex are above and below the cortical plate. At about eighteen to twenty weeks, thalamic afferents invade the deep zone of the cortical plate, synapses increase in density, and differentiation of cortical plate neurons commences (Molliver, Kostovic, & Vander Loos, 1973). This

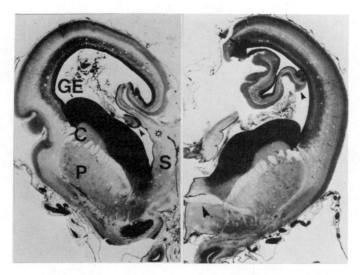

Fig. 11. Photomicrographs of 14 week human fetal brain taken in
          the frontal plane. On the left axons of hippocampal
          (small arrowhead) and neocortical pyramidal neurons ap-
          proach and cross the midline in a specialized region
          above the septal nuclei (S). At a slightly more caudal
          level on the right, the anterior commissure (large ar-
          rowhead) is already well developed. Germinal cells of
          the massive ganglionic eminence (GE) give rise to neu-
          rons of the caudate (C) and putamen (P). (Iron Hema-
          toxylin, 25X).

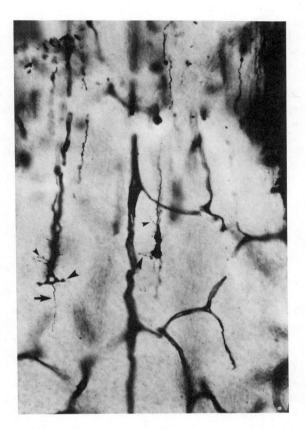

Fig. 12.   Photomicrograph of pyramidal neurons in the depths of
            the cortical plate in a human fetus of 18 weeks gesta-
            tion. The nucleus of the cell on the left is visible as
            a clear space, its apical shaft is observed somewhat by
            a contiguous blood vessel, and an axon exits from its
            base (arrow). Both pyramidal neurons exhibit early dif-
            ferentiation of their basilar dendrites (large arrow-
            heads) and the oblique branches of the apical shaft
            (small arrowheads). (Rapid Golgi, 250X).

is illustrated in Figure 12. (To date the cues which trigger this sequence of developmental events are largely unknown.)

The unequal forces generated by the differential development of inner and outer cortical layers cause its surface to buckle, and likely account for the convolutional pattern that character- izes the brain of humans and other higher mammals (Richman, Stewart, Hutchinson, & Caviness, 1975). The areas of primary sen- sory and motor thalamocortical projection exhibit the most preco- cious cell and fiber differentiation, and it is here that the first sulci and gyri appear about twenty-four weeks gestation (Marin-Padilla, 1970; Chi, Dooling, & Gilles, 1977). This is shown in Figure 13. As the gradient of cellular differentiation spreads outward from these primary zones, the buckling frequency of the cortical surface increases progressively, so that by birth at forty weeks gestation the gyral pattern of the human brain, as can be seen in Figure 14, is already well established.

ABNORMAL DEVELOPMENT OF THE CEREBRAL CORTEX

Many of the stages of cortical development are under genetic control and may fail subsequent to genetic mutation (Caviness & Rakic, 1978). The cerebral neocortex also appears to be particu- larly vulnerable to the pathological processes which strike during the developmental epoch. The remarkable complexity of events through which this organ develops, its large size and the long duration of its developmental cycle may be only the most obvious factors which confer a heightened vulnerability to disturbances of the maternal support system, infection, hydrocephalus and a host of other less well understood disease processes.

Developmental disorders of the human nervous system are often classified according to the epoch when the pathological process was judged to have occurred (Lemire et al., 1975). As discussed in the preceeding section, the stages of cerebral cortical devel- opment are continuous and overlapping, and include neurogenesis (6-16 weeks gestation); histogenesis; that is, the events through which cells are assembled into individual tissue components (8-20 weeks gestation) and, the stage of neuronal growth and differenti- ation, including synaptogenesis (18 weeks gestation to maturity). Pathological processes occuring during the stages of neurogenesis and histogenesis usually result in cortical malformations. The terms used traditionally to identify these malformations are de- scriptive only. The epochal classification has the virtue of es- tablishing a time during gestation when the pathologic process was maximally active, but neither the epochal nor the descriptive classifications necessarily conveys any information regarding causes or pathological process.

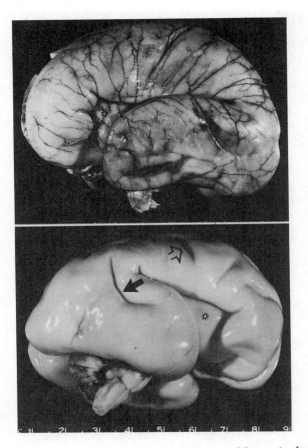

Fig. 13.   Lateral views of the brain from a 20 week (upper) and 24
           week old (lower) human fetus, respectively. Although
           the brain of the 20 week old fetus is swollen and dis-
           colored from terminal pathologic neurons, its cerebral
           surface is essentially smooth. The insular region (*)
           is not covered yet by the developing terminal lobe.   In
           the 24 week old fetus, the central (open arrow) and su-
           perior temporal sulci (arrow) are among the first to de-
           velop.

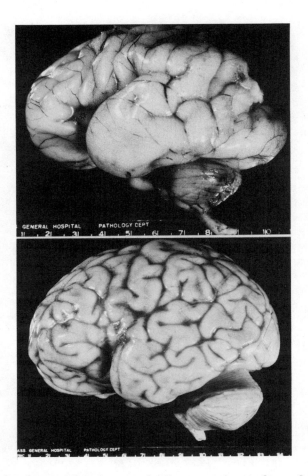

Fig. 14.   Left lateral views of the cerebrum from fetuses of 30
           (upper) and 40 (lower) weeks gestation. In the 30 week
           fetus, gyration has progressed in the central region and
           parasagittal convexity. Cortex of the anterior frontal
           and temporal areas is less convoluted. The insula (*)
           is still exposed. In the term infant, by contrast, gy-
           ration is far advanced and the insular region is
           covered.

In the following discussion, we will use the descriptive terms by which cortical malformations are commonly known, and will estimate the epoch from which each was judged to have arisen. In some instances, the topographic distribution of the lesion, and the quality of histological reaction, also suggest clues about potential pathological mechanisms. This approach has the advantage of generating theories of etiology and pathogenesis which can be tested experimentally or epidemiologically.

Disorders of Neurogenesis and Histogenesis

Anencephaly. (Virtually the entire forebrain, as well as varying portions of the brainstem and cerebellum, are absent (Lemire, Beckwith, & Warkany, 1978). This malformation is more commonly encountered in the miscarried or stillborn infant (Creasy & Alberman, 1976). It has been produced in experimental analysis by teratologic agents directed against the generative epithelium, resulting in failure of the anterior neural tube to close. Cerebral neurogenesis and histogenesis are initiated normally, but tissue contiguous to the site where the neural tube should have closed proliferates abnormally, displacing the adjacent forebrain. Ultimately, the entire forebrain becomes necrotic and degenerates. A variety of cytotoxic agents directed against the human fetus at the end of the first month of gestation, when neural tube closure should occur, probably cause this malformation in man.

Holoprosencephaly. This is a rare malformation of the rostral forebrain. Olfactory structures are invariably absent, and the eyes are variably malformed. One of the most severe examples of this malformation is associated with a single malformed eye, accounting for the descriptive term "cyclopia." There is a single cerebral cavity or ventricle surrounded by a shield-like shell of cortex which may be convoluted. This is shown in Figure 15. The cortex may be normally thick with a six layered pattern. In some cases, Yakovlev (1959) was able to identify several characteristic cytoarchitectural subfields. The horseshoe-shaped posterior rim of the cerebral vesicle consists of symmetrical hippocampal formations. Cortex with cytoarchitecture characteristic of the primary visual area is often present bilaterally and connected to the lateral geniculate bodies by a prominent myelinated fiber bundle, the optic radiation. In favorable specimens, Yakovlev found that the single anterior gyrus had no distinct layer IV and contained giant pyramids in layer V, a cytoarchitecture typical of the primary motor cortex. Neocortex of temporal and parietal areas was present bilaterally but reduced in volume, and the prefrontal areas were entirely absent. The thalamus and hypothalamus are usually malformed also, and the basal ganglia may be fused in the midline. It is as though the sector of the rostral neural tube which is normally the origin of structures forming the an-

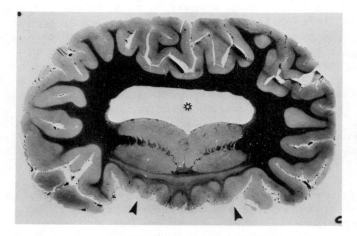

Fig. 15.   Frontal section stained for myelinated axons through the
            cerebrum of a child with holoprosenscephaly. There is a
            single ventricular cavity (*) surrounded by convoluted
            cortex of normal thickness. Insular cortex (arrowheads)
            is located in an anomalous ventral position (beneath)
            the basal ganglia which are fused in the midline.

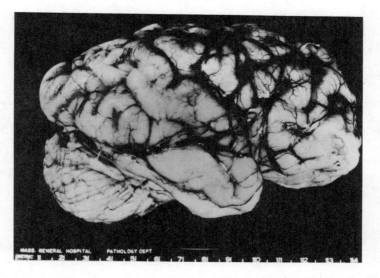

Fig. 16. Right lateral view of the brain of a 14 year old with microcephaly. The brain weighed 480 gms., less than half normal expected for age. The bulk of the parietal and frontal lobes is greatly reduced, and the gyral pattern is simplified.

terior-medial wall of the two cerebral vesicles had been destroyed, and continuity between the remaining portions re-established
in some way. Consistent with the view that the malformation is
caused primarily by a destructive process, is the observation that
the anterior diencephalon is replaced by a vascular fibroglial
scar. A similar malformation has been produced experimentally in
lower vertebrates by a variety of teratogens (Friede, 1975).

Holoprosencephaly must result from an abnormality of neurogenesis at the rostral end of the neural tube occurring after
closure of the anterior neuropore, but before evagination of pair-
ed cerebral vesicles; that is, between four and six weeks gestation. Most cases are sporadic, but a few are seen in association
with chromosomal disorders, such as trisomy 15. Most are stillborn, and survival beyond the first few years of life is exceptional. The severity of craniofacial deformities is variable.
Typical cases are profoundly retarded with epilepsy and spastic
weakness of the extremities.

Microcephally. Microcephally or true microencephaly desig-
nates a malformation in which brain weight and head circumference
are more than three deviations below the mean for age. The small-
ness of the head and brain are often in striking disproportion to
the face and body as a whole. The brainstem and cerebellum are
more normal in size and gross appearance. On neuropathologic examination the cerebral hemispheres are small and the convolutional
pattern simplified. This is demonstrated in Figure 16.

Abnormalities of cortical cytoarchitecture vary from mild to
severe. In some cases, the cerebral cortex is thin and the
laminar pattern is severely disordered (Robain & Lyon, 1972). Collections of neurons in heterotopic subcortical position may also
be present. In other cases, cortical thickness and cytoarchitecture are nearly normal, especially in the primary sensory and mot-
or areas, but there is an abnormal accentuation of the columnar
pattern, especially as shown in Figure 17, in the superficial
layers (Halperin, Williams, & Kolodny, 1982). Closer inspection
discloses that some radial columns are normally cellular, but are
accentuated by adjacent ones which are cell poor. The size of
individual neurons and the complexity of their dendritic arbors
appear normal in Golgi impregnations. By implication, microcephaly represents a failure of normal neurogenesis, especially of
later generated cells destined for neocortical association areas
and the outer cortical layers. The pathologic process must occur
relatively late in cortical cytogenesis, presumably around fourteen to sixteen weeks gestation.

In most cases, the etiology of microcephaly is not known.
Although familial cases are reported (Kloepfer, Platon & Hansche,
1964), the majority are sporadic. Similar malformations have been

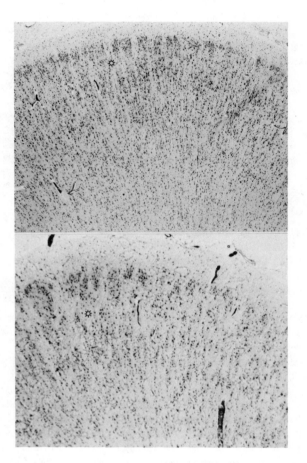

Fig. 17.   Photomicrographs of neocortex from the prefrontal (upper
           and superior temporal (lower) cortical regions of the
           child with microcephaly. The normal six layered cyto-
           architecture is relatively indistinct and the radially
           striate appearance is accentuated, more so in the
           superior temporal gyrus, owing to the presence of hypo-
           cellular columns (*), especially in layers II-IV.
           (Cresyl violet, upper 48X, lower 64X).

produced in animals by radiation damage or the administration of mitotic poisons (Riggs, McGrath, & Schwarz, 1956; Wisniewski, Haddad, Rabe, Dumas, & Shek, 1977). Microcephaly has also been reported in humans after radiation exposure (Dekaban, 1968). The degree of motor and intellectual handicap, and the incidence of associated epilepsy is in general proportional to the severity of the cytoarchitectural and other associated abnormalities. In cases where cytoarchitectural changes are minor, the acquisition of motor milestones may be nearly normal and intellectual impairment slight, even though the brain may be less than half normal size (Halperin et al., 1981; Dooling & Richardson, 1980).

Megalencephaly. Essentially the converse of microcephaly, megalencephaly refers to brains which are more than three standard deviations greater than the norm in weight. The gyral pattern may be normal or anomalously excessive (Friede, 1975). Cortical laminar pattern is usually normal, but subcortical heterotopias (see below) are occasionally present. Excessive brain size has been hypothesized to result from a greater than normal number of neurons and/ or glial cells in the brain, as well as to a greater than normal size of the individual cellular elements. Golgi analysis of cortical neurons in one case failed to confirm an abnormality of cell size (R.S. Williams, unpublished). To the extent that this observation is correct, the malformation may reflect abnormal control of cell numbers through the process of cell death. This process, essential to the fine regulation of the number of cells recruited into neuronal circuits (Jacobson, 1978), may be disordered by mechanisms which are completely unknown.

Disorders of commissuration. Defects of commissuration may be total; that is, absence of anterior, hippocampal and callosal commissures, or partial and involve only the posterior portions of the corpus callosum. Figure 18 illustrates this condition. Most cases probably represent a partial developmental failure owing to a pathologic process, genetic or acquired, occurring after fourteen weeks gestation. When the defect is restricted to the corpus callosum, the anterior commissure may be abnormally large, suggesting that fibers destined initially for the corpus callosum may have taken an alternative path. The cerebral hemispheres usually appear normal along the lateral convexity, but the gyral pattern of the medial surface is abnormal with a radial or spoke-like configuration. Abnormalities of commissuration may occur alone, or in association with cytoarchitectural changes of varying severity and subcortical heterotopias.

When the cut surface of the brain is viewed in the frontal plane, the lateral ventricles appear enlarged, and a stump of white matter tissue extends medially below the cingulate gyrus. The fornix, a myelinated fiber bundle connecting the hippocampus with the rostral forebrain, is suspended in normal position from

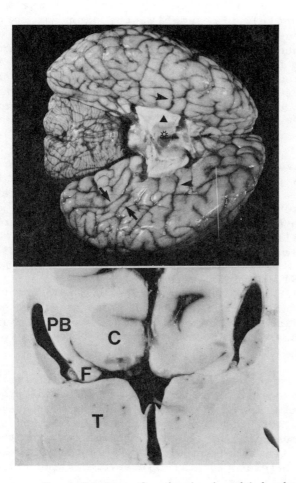

Fig. 18. Upper: Dorsal view of a brain in which the corpus cal-
          losum is absent. The cerebral hemispheres fall apart
          exposing the third ventricle (*) and diencephalon (tri-
          angle). On the medial occipital surface, the configu-
          ration of the calcarine and parieto-occipital sulci
          (arrows) is normal, but at the medial edge of the cere-
          bral hemispheres the gyral pattern has an anomalous
          radial configuration (arrowheads). Lower: Coronal sec-
          tion of the formalin fixed brain at the level of the
          thalamus (T). Stumps of white matter tissue (PB), an
          anomalous longitudinal fiber bundle, extend medially
          under the cingulate gyrus (C). The fornix (F) is sus-
          pended from the medial edge of PB.

the medial edge of the white matter stump. Microscopically the stump consists of a longitudinal bundle of myelinated fibers (Probst's bundle). Presumably, the axons of cortical neurons seeking interhemispheric connections arrived at the midline normally, and when unable to cross, coursed instead longitudinally as the anomalous fiber bundle. The persistence of this bundle after birth and throughout the life of the individual is convincing evidence that its axons formed anomalous alternative synaptic connections with neuronal groups elsewhere in the same hemisphere. The precise nature of these anomalous circuits, almost surely cortico-cortical, is still unknown.

Most cases of callosal agenesis are sporadic, but familial occurrence is recorded and it occurs also with a variety of congenital anomaly syndromes (Friede, 1975). In isolated cases the clinical picture is highly variable ranging from no apparent abnormality to profound mental retardation with epilepsy (Ehlinger, Blakemore, Miller, & Wilson, 1974). In general, the degree of neurologic impairment is proportional to the severity of associated cerebral abnormalities, such as heterotopias (Loeser & Alvord, 1968), but intellectual impairment and epilepsy may occur even when callosal agenesis and Probst's bundle are the only malformation identified. Perhaps in these cases the anomalous circuitry established by the longitudinal callosal bundle impairs normal cerebral function and lowers the threshold for seizure activity.

Disorders of neuronal migration. The migratory mechanism is fragile and susceptible to injury by pathological processes striking at any time between eight and eighteen to twenty weeks gestation. Neurons arrested in migration may survive and differentiate, presumably sustained by synaptic connections with their neighbors and perhaps with other cortical and subcortical structures as well. These heterotopias may take several forms (Friede, 1975).

1.   **Cerebral heterotopias.** *Nodular heterotopias* are conglomerate masses of neurons, usually adjacent to the ventricular surface and surrounded by a shell of myelinated fibers. This is illustrated in Figure 19. They are more prevalent in the posterior half of the hemisphere, especially under the dorso-lateral convexity. On microscopic inspection, individual nodular heterotopias contain differentiated neurons, including pyramidal and non-pyramidal cells. In many instances, an internal cellular organization is evident. In general, larger pyramids are more peripheral and successively smaller ones more centrally placed. In favorable sections, the apicies of many pyramidal neurons seem to be oriented toward the center of the nodule. The central zone consists of a feltwork of poorly myelinated fibers and few cells, and is hence structurally similar to a molecular layer (Dooling & Richardson, 1980).

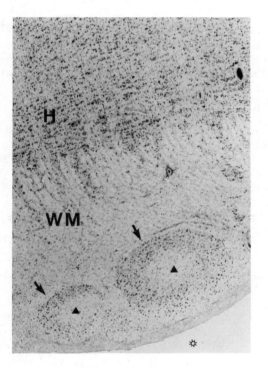

Fig. 19. Nodular heterotopias (arrows) are encapsulated by mye-
          linated axons of the white matter (WM) adjacent to the
          ventricular surface (*).   Larger pyramidal and small
          non-pyramidal neurons are organized to the periphery of
          the nodular heterotopia and oriented toward a fiber rich
          cell poor central zone (triangles).   These nodular
          heterotopias are from the brain of an 8 month old agyric
          infant.   Presumably they developed in-situ in the
          germinal epithelium, and never began migration on radial
          glial fibers.   H represents a broad field of heterotopic
          neurons which were arrested in the course of their mi-
          gration. (Cresyl Violet,40X) (see Fig. 21).

Heterotopias may also be organized into a laminar zone in the central white matter (Friede, 1975). *Laminar heterotopias* are also more prevalent in the posterior hemisphere. Microscopic inspection reveals a variety of differentiated pyramidal and nonpyramidal neurons, and pyramids are oriented radially with their apical shafts oriented toward the overlying cortex.

Presumably, the abnormality causing nodular and laminar heterotopias occurs after neurogenesis, but before migrating neurons have achieved their final cortical destinations. Nodular periventricular heterotopias are probably composed of neurons which differentiated *in situ*, and were never entrained normally by the migratory processes.

Nodular and laminar heterotopias may be seen as small localized malformations in relative isolation, in which case the overlying cortex may be of nearly normal thickness and cytoarchitecture. In some instances, the overlying cortex has a prominent columnar appearance as described above for microcephally. Subcortical heterotopias may also be seen in association with other malformations, such as agenesis of corpus callosum, agyria and malformations of the cerebellum.

2. **Agyria and pachygyria.** When the disorder of neuronal migration is more severe and widespread there are also changes, as illustrated in Figure 20, in the surface appearance of the overlying cortex. The brain is small and its surface is relatively smooth or *agyric*. There may also be reduced numbers of abnormally broad or *pachygyric* convolutions (Stewart, Richman, & Caviness, 1975). With few exceptions, the cortical malformation exhibits a striking regional topography, being maximally severe along the lateral convexities of the parietal, occipital and temporal lobes. The gyral pattern of the ventral and medial cortical surfaces is more normal in appearance.

The microscopic appearance of the malformed cerebral wall is also characteristic, and four zones are classically described. The outermost is a thin, cell poor zone continuous with and comparable to the molecular layer of normal cortex. Second is a cellular zone representing the incompletely formed true cortex. The true cortex is separated from a broad field of heterotopic neurons by a narrow hypocellular band. As one proceeds from agyric to pachygyric and to normally convoluted areas, the thickness of the heterotopia decreases and that of the true cortex increases proportionally.

By implication, development proceeded normally until the fourth fetal month when a pathologic process caused an abrupt, nearly complete arrest of further neuronal migration from a restricted region of the ventricular germinal zone (Stewart et al.,

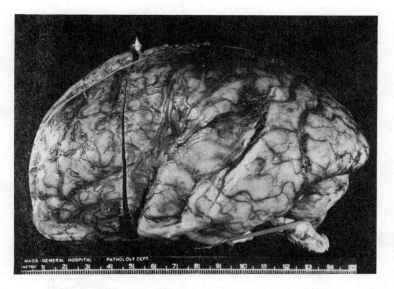

Fig. 20.   Left lateral view of an agyric brain from a 14 year old
           child (a cut has been made through the frontal lobes).
           Short shallow sulci are present along the lateral con-
           vexity of the frontal and temporal lobes, but much of
           the brain surface is smooth.

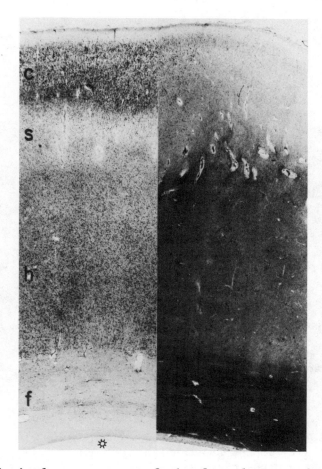

Fig. 21. Typical appearance of the four layers of the agyric
cerebral wall as seen in stains for cells (left) and
myelinated axons (right). A cell sparse zone, perhaps
representing a glial scar (S), separates the incompletely formed true cortex (C) from a broad field of
heterotopic neurons (H) arrested in migration. A small
fascicle of myelinated fibers (F) separates the heterotopia from the ventricular surface (*).

1975). Heterotopic neurons are seen also in the medulla and cerebellum, structures which are developing by long distance neuronal migration at about the same time. In most instances, the etiology of agyria is unknown. Exceptionally it is seen in siblings, suggesting the action of a mutant gene (Dieker, Edwards, & Zurhein, 1969). However, its unique topography is congruent with the distal fields of perfusion of the major cerebral vessels, suggesting that it may arise from arterial perfusion failure (Stewart et al., 1975). These arterial zones are established well in advance of when the malformation is judged to have occured (Van der Eecken, 1969), but to date, there is not direct evidence to support this hypothesis.

When agyric cortex is examined in rapid Golgi impregnations, remarkable insights into the range of neuronal plasticity in the human brain emerge. Figures 22 and 23 demonstrate these findings. In most instances the findings are in accord with cytologic analyses of cortical malformations in experimental animals (Pinto-Lord & Caviness, 1979). Whether in appropriate cortical or anomalous subcortical position, the full range of pyramidal and non-pyramidal neurons are identifiable and have well developed dendritic arbors. Those which are normally spine rich are invested richly with spines of normal morphology. Evidently then, these class characteristic attributes of neuronal phenotype develop independently of positional cues, and are presumably under control of the genome. In the true cortex, neurons of the same class are aligned tangentially, roughly comparable to layers III through VI in the normal. The true cortex appears to be particularly deficient in small neurons found normally in layers II through IV. In the heterotopia, neurons are not organized by class into discrete tangential laminae, but appear to be distributed randomly. In both true cortex and the heterotopia, pyramidal neurons are aligned normally orthogonal to the cerebral surface, but in the true cortex, many pyramids are inverted 180 degrees in polarity. Their apical dendrites descend away from the surface. Axons of pyramidal neurons arise normally from the inferior pole, but the axon of inverted pyramidal usually emerges anomalously from the proximal portion of the apical dendritic shaft. The normal alignment of pyramidal neurons in either cortical or heterotopic subcortical position suggests that their unique relationship with the radial glial fibers is sufficient to insure proper alignment when differentiation occurs at any point along the migratory trajectory. The configuration of inverted pyramids in the true cortex suggests that their axon developed normally from the inferior pole during the course of migration, and that the apical dendrite also has the option of arising from the inferior pole, perhaps in response to a shift in trophic environmental cues. The observation that neurons of the true cortex are organized by class into recognizable sublaminae, and those of the heterotopia are not, confirms that lamination occurs only if successively younger cells are delivered in

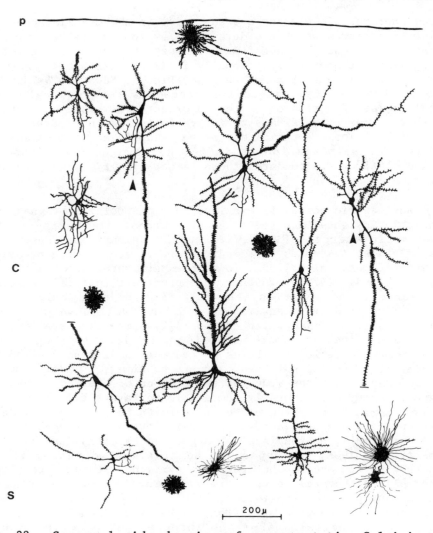

Fig. 22.   Camera lucida drawing of representative Golgi impreg-
           nated neurons and astrocytes from the true cortex (C)
           and cell sparse zone (S) of the agyric brain. Pyramidal
           and nonpyramidal neurons have well developed dendritic
           arbors, and those which are normally spine-rich are in-
           vested richly with spines. Pyramidal neurons are
           aligned radially orthogonal to the cortical surface (P),
           but two are inverted in polarity with downwardly di-
           rected dendrites. The axon of properly oriented pyrami-
           dal cells exits normally from their base, whereas the
           axons of inverted pyramids exit from the proximal apical
           shaft (arrowheads). The apical shafts of properly ori-
           ented medium to large pyramidal cells located anoma-
           lously subjacent to the surface must turn to course
           tangentially.

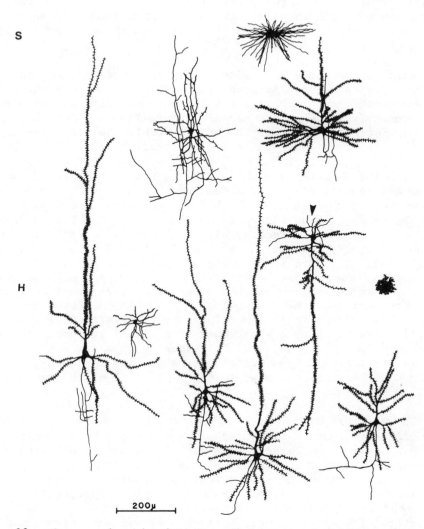

S

H

200μ

Fig. 23.   Camera lucida drawing of representative neurons and
astrocytes from the heterotopia (H) of lissencephaly.
Like neurons of the true cortex, heterotopic neurons
have developed class characteristic dendritic and
axonal features.   Pyramidal neurons are normally aligned
and most are properly oriented with their apical shafts
ascending toward the cerebral surface.   In contrast to
the inverted pyramids in Figure 22, the axon of the inverted pyramid illustrated here in the heterotopic zone
exits normally from the base of the cell (arrowhead),
but then recurves to descend toward the subcortical
white matter.

normal sequence into the cortical plate. This suggests that although neurons with the same birthdate ultimately arrive at the same destination, their rates of migration may be very unequal in the human brain.

Although infants born with agyria may appear normal initially, the clinical course is predictable, and to some extent, rather characteristic. The head fails to grow normally and psychomotor development is profoundly retarded. Typically, infantile spasms and a chaotically abnormal EEG appear within the first few months of life. Few survive beyond the first year.

3. **The Zellweger malformation.** This disorder, a complex systemic metabolic disorder associated with abnormal brain development, is transmitted by autosomal recessive inheritance (Volpe & Adams, 1972). There is an abnormality, illustrated in Figure 24, in the surface gyral pattern which occurs bilaterally around the central sulcus and Sylvian fissure (Evrard, Caviness, & Lyon, 1978). The gyri in the Sylvian region are smaller than normal, whereas those more medially in the central region appear wider. The cell pattern of the cortex is also abnormal, especially in the region of the gyral anomaly. This is illustrated in Figure 25. Although the five principal cellular layers are explicitly present, they are narrower than normal and contain a reduced complement of cells. Cell poor columns are also present. This is particularly true of the most superficial layers, a disparity which is accentuated in the broad gyri of the central region.

In this respect, the cortical anomaly bears a superficial resemblance to that of lissencephaly and microcephaly. Unlike the latter, however, a large contingent of neurons is distributed in heterotopic position throughout all levels of the cortex and extending deeply into the subcortical white matter. Among the neurons in heterotopic position are cells of all morphological classes: that is, cells which are normally destined for all of the neocortical layers. The cell pattern analysis suggests that the malformation is a consequence of a disorder of a migration which is partial in degree; that is, it effects only a limited proportion of neurons, but extends throughout the entire period of migration (Evrard et al., 1978). The pathologic process appears to extend also into the stage of growth and differentiation, as evidenced by a generalized proliferation of astrocytes and abnormal myelination. Possibly, the general metabolic abnormality associated with the Zellweger mutation causes a non-specific disruption of cell metabolism which interferes with the ability of cells to migrate. Alternatively, the mutation may target more specifically upon some aspect of the mechanism which permits neurons to ascend normally along the radial glial fiber.

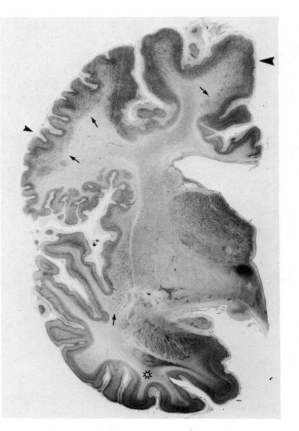

Fig. 24. Hemi-frontal section of the cerebral hemisphere at the level of the midthalamus from a child with the Zellweger malformation. Gyral width and cortical thickness are increased dorso-medially (large arrowhead), and decreased laterally (small arrowhead). Heterotopic neurons are scattered within and subjacent to the abnormally convoluted cortex (arrows). By contrast, the thickness and convolutional pattern of neo-cortex in the medial and ventral temporal area (*) is more normal, and there are fewer heterotopic neurons (Cresyl violet, 2X).

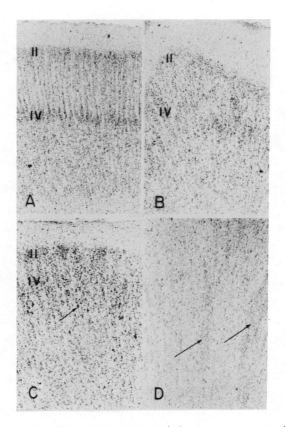

Fig. 25.   Neocortex in the normal (A), microgyric (B) and pachy-
           gyric (C) regions of the Zellweger brain. Roman numer-
           als II and IV are at levels of corresponding cortical
           layers. The arrow in C indicates a large pyramidal neu-
           ron typical of those (Betz) encountered normally in
           layer V of the motor cortex. The arrows in D point to
           clusters of heterotopic neurons subjacent to the pachy-
           gyric cortex. These neurons are small "granular" cells,
           typical of those found normally in layer IV of primary
           sensory and associational cortices. (Cresyl Violet,
           68X).

4.   **Driftwood cortex.** This malformation, apparently transmitted also by autosomal recessive inheritance, is unique among
malformations in man in that large axon fascicles are directed to
the most superficial plane of the cortex, imparting a "driftwood"
appearance (Rebeiz, Wolf, & Adams, 1968). In this respect, at
least, driftwood cortex in man is similar to the reeler neocortical malformation in mice, which also occurs consequent to autosomal
recessive mutation (Caviness & Rakic, 1978). In the mutant mouse,
the abnormality of axon trajectory appears very early as the cortical plate emerges. Its mechanism is unknown, and the developmental history of the human malformation is also unknown.

5.   **Extracerebral ectopias.** A heterogeneous group of cerebral malformations may be associated with neuronal ectopias; that
is, neural masses located within the meningeal space, extrinsic to
the cerebral hemisphere (Caviness et al., 1978a,b). This anomaly
has been associated with the "fetal alcohol" syndrome (Jones,
Smith, Ulleland, & Streissgath, 1973), but is probably not specific to any teratogeny.

The illustrated example in Figure 26 is associated with what
appears to have been a relatively mild injury directed to the most
superficial part of the developing cortex; that is, to the inter-
face of the mesenchymal membranes and the molecular layer. At
points where damage has occurred, a mesenchymal-neuroglial scar
has formed. Young neurons, presumably already in position at the
most superficial level of the cortex when the injury occurred,
have apparently resumed their migrations subsequent to the event.
Many have migrated beyond the limits of the central nervous system
to establish a large colony of neural cells in the subarachnoid
compartment. This malformation in many ways underscores the critical role of the molecular layer, and pial-glial membrane, as factors constraining the positions of young neurons at the end of
migration.

Disorders Arising During the Period of Neuronal Growth and Differentiation

In the preceeding section, cerebral abnormalities resulting
from pathologic processes active during the first half of gestation were discussed. Other characteristic malformations, or perhaps more appropriately "deformations," occur in the second half
of gestation, during the period of growth and differentiation of
neurons and their supporting tissues.

Polymicrogyria. Polymicrogyria is a cerebral malformation
characterized by excessive surface convolution and abnormal cytoarchitecture. Similar to agyria, polymicrogyria usually exhibits
a unique regional topography with the malformation maximum para-
sagittally along the lateral convexity. This is shown in Figure

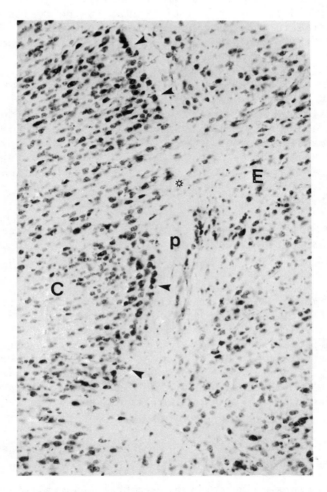

Fig. 26. A bridge of neurons and glial tissue (*) extends between cortex (C) and the extracortical neuroglial extopia (E). The pia (p) is intact adjacent to the bridge. Neurons of the cortex adjacent to the bridge have taken up the space normally occupied by fibers of the molecular layer (arrowheads). (Cresyl Violet, 165X).

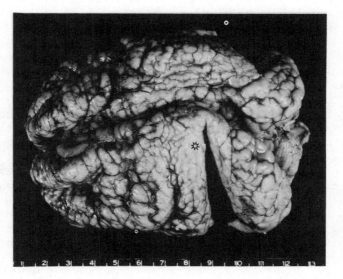

Fig. 27.   Dorsal view of a brain with polymicrogyria as seen after
           formalin fixation. The frontal lobes are in the left,
           and the cerebellum can be seen behind the occipital
           lobes to the right. The cobblestone appearance of poly-
           microgyric cortex is maximum in the posterior parasagit-
           tal convexity where the cortex is greatly thinned, so
           much so that it has partially collapsed (*). Cortex of
           the frontal pole is more normally convoluted.

27. Cortex of the ventral and medial surfaces is more normally
convoluted with a six layered cytoarchitecture. As classically
described, the malformed cortex is abnormally thin and contains
four principal layers, as illustrated in Figure 28 (Richman,
Stewart, & Caviness, 1974). The first layer of the abnormal cortex is a plexiform zone continuous with, and comparable to, the
molecular layer of adjacent normal cortex. Although excessively
undulating, the cytoarchitecture of the second polymicrogyric
layer shares many similarities with laminae II through IV of the
normal cortex, with which it is also continuous (see Figure 2).
Polymicrogyric layer 2 is separated from layer 4 by a thin cell
poor zone which is a glial scar continuous with midcortical layers
of adjacent normal cortex. Subcortical heterotopic neurons are
not typically found. The unequal development of neurons in the
outer and inner tiers of the abnormally thin cortex results in an
excessive buckling frequency (Richman et al., 1975), hence the
term polymicrogyria.

Polymicrogyria appears to result from a destructive pathologic process affecting neocortex in restricted topographic fashion at a stage after neuronal migration is largely complete, but
before the formation of primary gyri and sulci; that is, between
twenty and thirty weeks gestation. This hypothesis, based on morphologic criteria, is sustained by the observation of polymicrogyria in the offspring of mothers exposed to carbon monoxide at mid-
gestation (Bankl & Jellinger, 1967). Although the etiology in
many cases is obscure, polymicrogyria may be seen after intrauterine infection with toxoplasmosis or cytomegalovirus (Friede,
1975).

Neurological abnormalities vary in proportion to the extent
of the cerebral malformation. Small foci of symmetrical polymicrogyria may be an incidental finding postmorten in people judged
to be normal neurologically. When extensive, the brain is generally small and the history includes profound psychomotor retardation and epilepsy. The glial scar encountered at midcortical
levels isolates the outer regions of the cortex from the rest of
the brain (Williams, Ferrante, & Caviness, 1976). Presumably neurons of the outer layers survive and are sustained by the elabora-
tion of anomalous local circuits. This is shown in Figure 29.
These anomalous circuits could be expected to facilitate the tangential spread of abnormal electrical activity, and may explain
the high incidence of paroxysmal abnormalities seen typically in
EEG's of individuals with this malformation (Caviness & Williams,
1979).

Porencephaly. The second half of gestation is also a time of
active gliogenesis, and the competence of young astrocytes to form
a dense glial scar is probably not well established until after
thirty weeks gestation (Williams et al., 1976). Polymicrogyria

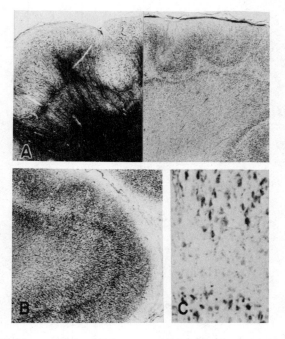

Fig. 28.   A.   Adjacent sections stained for myelinated axons
           (left) and cells (right) showing the four layers of
           classical polymicrogyric cortex. B. An area of transi-
           tion (*) between polymicrogyric cortex (left) and normal
           cortex (right), confirming that the cell sparse third
           microgyric layer is continuous with mid-cortical layers
           in the normal. C. Higher power view of the cell sparse
           zone demonstrating that it contains predominantly astro-
           cytes and very few neurons.

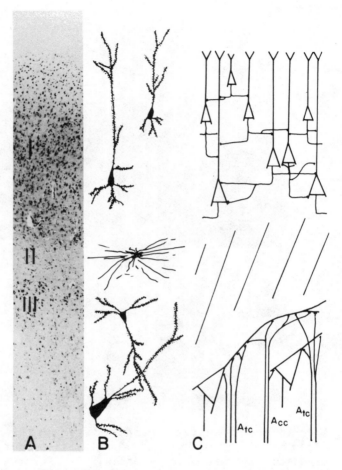

Fig. 29. A. Photomicrograph of polymicrogyric cortex as seen
          with a cresyl violet stain. Roman numerals designate
          the three cellular zones. B. Representative neurons as
          drawn from Golgi impregnations. A fibrous astrocyte
          marks the glial scar at the level of cell destruction.
          C. Schematic model of presumed synaptic organization of
          polymicrogyric cortex. There may be a proliferation of
          axon collaterals among tier I neurons above the scar,
          and below the scar a tangentially oriented pyramidal
          cell is contacted by several groups of thalamocortical
          afferents (Atc) and by corticocortical afferents
          (Acc).

likely results from a subtotal destructive process causing cell loss, meager gliosis and subsequent tissue distortion. When the destructive process is more severe, large defects occur in the cerebral wall.

Polyencephaly refers to focal cerebral defects due to destructive processes occurring early in the second half of gestation. Most are bilateral and relatively symmetrical. This can be noted in Figure 30. The defect is covered by a translucent glial-mesenchymal membrane. Polymicrogyric cortex may border the walls of the defect, but most of the surviving cortex is usually normal. Porencephalic defects typically occur in zones perfused by the major cerebral arteries (Myers, Valerio, Martin, & Nelson, 1973; Levine, Fisher, & Caviness, 1974). Depending upon their size and location, they may be associated with intellectual impairment, cerebral palsy and epilepsy.

Hydranencephaly. Hydranencephaly is another malformation resulting from a destructive process occurring around mid-gestation (Halsey, Allen, & Chamberlan, 1971). In severe cases, virtually the entire cerebral cortex, as illustrated in Figure 31, may be destroyed and replaced by a translucent fibro-glial membrane. More typically, the entire cerebrum anterior to the occipital, inferior parietal and inferior temporal lobes is destroyed completely. The remnants of posterior neocortex are usually normally convoluted with normal cytoarchitecture, but cortex at the border of the defect may be polymicrogyric. Although the area of destroyed cortex usually corresponds nicely to the territory of the internal carotid artery, and its anterior and middle cerebral intracranial branches, the basal ganglia which also receive their blood supply from the middle cerebral artery are usually normal histologically. In support of an ischemic process causing this malformation in man is the observation that similar malformations are produced in experimental animals, including fetal monkeys (Myers, 1969), after occlusion of the carotid arteries at mid-gestation. Nevertheless, the etiology in most human cases is obscure. In a few instances, cerebral arteriograms confirmed slender but intact intracranial vessels, but there are no published reports of pathological examination of the carotid arteries.

Children with hydranencephaly may appear normal at birth, but fail to achieve normal milestones. Head circumference may be enlarged at birth, but more typically enlarges at an accelerated rate post-natally. The diagnosis is often made clinically by a characteristic pattern of cranial trans-illumination, as shown in Figure 32.

Ulegyria and cerebral cortical sclerosis. When the cerebral cortex is subjected to destructive processes such as intrauterine

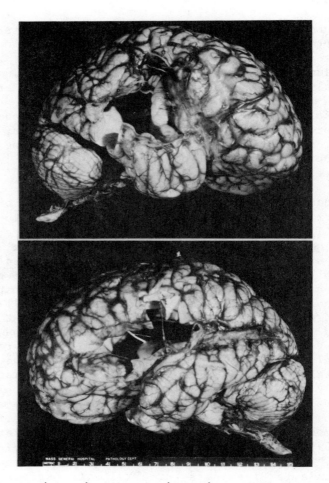

Fig. 30.   Right (upper) and left (lower) lateral views of a poren-
           cephalic brain after formalin fixation. (Several tissue
           blocks have been removed from the edge of the defect.)
           Cortex at the edge of the cerebral defect has a hyper-
           convoluted, microgyric appearance. The convolutional
           pattern of the remainder of the brain is normal. In the
           lower figure small isolated strands of white matter, all
           of the internal capsule, bridge the isolated cortex
           above and the brainstem below.

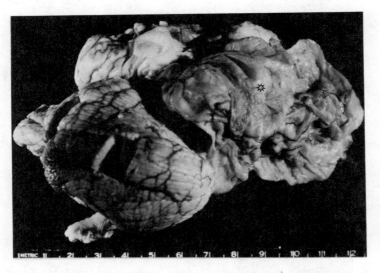

Fig. 31. Right lateral view of an hydraencephalic brain with a normal appearing cerebellum to the left (a wedge of tissue has been removed from the cerebellum). The cerebrum is replaced, virtually entirely, by a collapsed fibro-glial membrane (*).

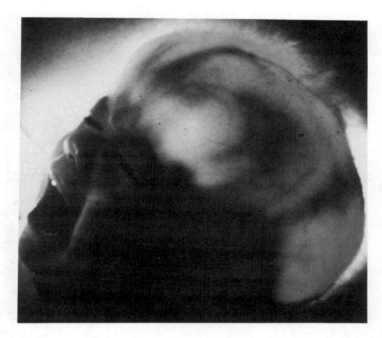

Fig. 32.   Abnormal cranial trans-illumination typical of that seen
in cases of hydranencephaly. In a darkened room a light
is placed behind the head, and in the absence of intervening normal brain tissue the fluid filled cavity
transmits light.

hypoxia-ischemia after thirty weeks gestation, tissue necrosis is associated with an increasing capacity for glial proliferation and scar tissue formation, or sclerosis. Normally formed gyri which are injured become shrunken and firm, imparting an abnormality of surface convolution called *ulegyria*. Figures 33 and 34 illustrate this process. Although they are superficially similar, ulegyria is different histologically from polymicrogyria, and implies a pathologic process occurring much later in gestation.

DISCUSSION

As is evident from the preceding discussion, the causes for most of these human developmental disorders are still largely unknown. Infrequently, they are seen in association with chromosomal abnormalities or recur in families, suggesting a gene mutation; but even then the sequence of events leading to characteristic brain maldevelopment are largely undefined. These conceptual deficiencies underscore the fact that currently we understand the cellular events of brain development only in their broadest outlines; major questions are unresolved relating to their molecular mechanisms and genetic regulation. The study of human pathology, as demonstrated above, uniquely poses the relevant questions but answers relatively few. We are forced to rely heavily on analytical experiments conducted with laboratory animals. Unfortunately, there are currently very few genetic or teratologic paradigms appropriate for studying the pathology of neurogenesis and histogenesis in man (Caviness & Rakic, 1978). Therefore, new animal models must be devised. Particularly important themes for future study are the developmental mechanisms which control the number of cells in the central nervous system, which determine cell class, which assure cell migration along the radial glial fiber, which dictate cell positions in the cortex after migration is complete, and which orchestrate the interactions between developing dendrites and axons, leading to the formation of interneuronal circuits. The challenge is to develop and apply new methods designed to answer some of these questions. Improved techniques of tissue culture and cell separation, the ability to generate monoclonal antibodies toward specific cell surface antigens, and recent advances in lectin and immunocytochemistry promise to make such inquiries possible in the near future.

An impression gained repeatedly from the neuropathologic examination of human developmental disorders, such as those outlined above, is that many seem to arise secondary to acquired destructive processes. When an etiology can be defined, particularly for those arising during the second half of gestation, it is congenital infection or cerebral perfusion failure (Friede, 1975). Maternal hypoxia, diabetes, hypotension and hypertension, premature placental separation or excessive infarction, and premature de-

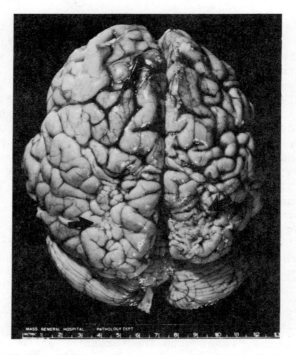

Fig. 33.   Dorsal view of the brain from a child with mental retar-
           dation and cerebral palsy illustrating shrunken, hyper-
           convoluted cortex in the parieto-occipital regions para-
           sagittally.   The hyper-convolution of ulegyria as
           illustrated here bears some superficial resemblance to
           that of polymicrogyria illustrated in Figure 26.

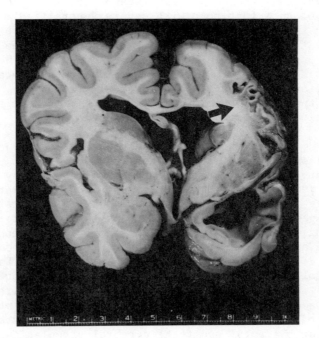

Fig. 34. Coronal section of the formalin fixed brain at the level
of the basal ganglia from a child with a history of
perinatal ischemic encephalopathy. The lateral convexity is ulegyric. As seen here, ulegyric cortex is
shrunken and gliosed, and includes necrosis of the
underlying white matter. The ventricals are enlarged,
presumably due to the reduction in tissue volume. This
appearance is typical of destructive neuropathologic
processes effecting the cerebrum late in gestation or in
the perinatal period.

livery are all known to be of potential significance in this regard. However, in almost half the cases of cerebral palsy, which
is classically attributed to cerebral ischemia, the available
clinical information does not suggest predisposing factors
(Christensen & Melchior, 1967).

A case reported recently by Adams, Prod'hom and Rabinowics
(1977), highlights the need for further research. They examined
the brain of an infant born with severe generalized hypotonia and
respiratory insufficiency. Death occurred a few hours after birth
and neuropathologic examination revealed widespread nerve cell
loss and a prominent inflammatory response, dating the pathology
to at least a week before birth. There was no evidence of congenital infection or placental pathology. In retrospect, the mother
was aware that fetal movement seemed less just prior to delivery,
but her health was judged to be excellent.

Experiments by Myers and associates (1975, 1979) using fetal
monkeys are of interest and potential significance in this regard.
They have developed surgical techniques whereby monkey fetuses can
be removed temporarily from the uterus while appropriate monitoring devices are applied, and returned to the uterus for the remainder of gestation. Later when pregnant monkeys are restrained
for testing, unanesthetized mothers become fearful and exhibit an
appropriate autonomic response. Although maternal blood pressure
and pulse rise appropriately, the cerebral circulation of the
fetus may fall substantially, sometimes to levels compatible with
tissue destruction. Placental and fetal cerebral circulation are
protected when the pregnant monkey is lightly anesthetized. Experiments of this type may provide new insights into the pathophysiology of placental and fetal cerebral circulation, which when
combined with improved antepartum care and non-invasive techniques
of fetal monitoring, could result in earlier detection and prevention of ischemic encephalopathies.

An even more distressing problem for the neuropathologist are
the 30% or so of moderately to severely retarded individuals whose
brains appear "normal" by conventional neuropathologic criteria
(Cavanagh, 1972). In general, brain weights are lower, but most
fall within two standard deviations of the mean. The implication
is that neurons are generated in sufficient numbers, are in their
proper postmigratory positions, grow and establish synaptic connections, but that critical steps in neuronal differentiation or
neuronal circuit organization fail late in gestation or early
postnatally. The result is a brain of near normal size and shape
which is nevertheless poorly equipped for normal perception, information processing and/or environmental interaction during critical postnatal stages of brain development.

The dilemma for the neuropathologist derives, at least in part, from the limitations of the methods available for morphologic analysis of brain tissue postmortem. Traditionally used routine cell and fiber stains have been employed for over one hundred years to assess cellular pattern and histologic reaction. However, as pointed out previously, most of the neuron, and particularly its receptive surfaces, are unstained by these methods.

Using the method of Golgi described previously, Purpura and colleagues (1974, 1979) have demonstrated convincingly in some cases that the pathological anatomy lies at the level of individual neurons and their dendritic processes. Neocortical pyramids, the normally spine-rich projection neurons, may have too few spines or spines which are distorted morphologically. This is demonstrated in Figure 35. Changes in spine density and morphology would be expected to substantially attenuate a large proportion of synaptic inputs to cortical pyramids. Changes in the density and morphology of dendritic spines have been produced in experimental animals by a variety of environmental manipulations (see Williams et al., 1980, for review). The significance of these findings as regards the pathophysiology of human mental retardation, however, is still poorly understood.

More recently, Purpura, Suzuki, Rapin and Wurzelmann (1980) have identified other cases in which the nerve cell pathology is characterized by varicose dilation of neuronal dendritic segments. Dendritic spines are also reduced in number. When examined with the electron microscope, the swollen dendritic segments contain mitochondria and abnormal accumulations of microfilaments, suggesting abnormalities of the structure and distribution of cytoskeletal proteins. This subgroup, of whom several examples have now been identified, share a similar clinical syndrome of psychomotor deterioration and epilepsy progressive in the first postnatal year.

Despite these important recent advances, cases are still encountered where convincing neuronal abnormalities are not apparent, even in Golgi preparations and electron micrographs (Huttenlocher, 1974; Cragg, 1975; Williams et al., 1980). These cases present a continuing challenge to the researcher interested in the pathophysiology of human developmental disorders.

Recent technological advances in the neurosciences are being adapted increasingly for application to the human brain, and hold great promise for expanding the frontiers of neuropathological investigation in the near future. For example, techniques are now available for quantitative analysis of dendritic arbors in Golgi impregnations of human brain (Buell & Coleman, 1979; Paldino & Purpura, 1980; Matthysse & Williams, 1980) and may provide new insights into changes in neuronal size or shape specific for cer-

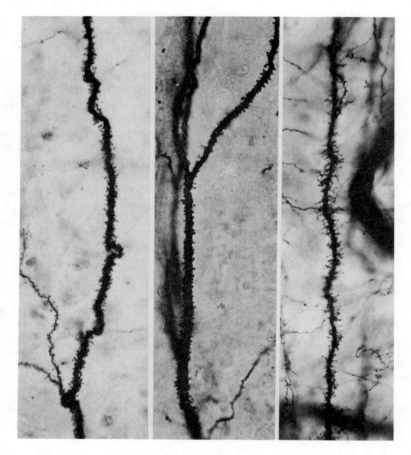

Fig. 35.   Photomicrographs of the apical dendritic shafts of layer
           V pyramidal neurons from a 5 year old child (left), and
           individuals with mental retardation (center and right).
           Normally pyramidal apical shafts are invested richly
           with spines measuring 1-3 microns in length.   In cases
           of mental retardation, spine density may be reduced
           (center), or spines may exhibit morphological abnormal-
           ities, such as the exceptionally long tortuous ones
           illustrated on the right. (Rapid Golgi, 800X).

tain disease states. In addition, it is now feasible to take small pieces of brain tissue obtained from humans at biopsy or postmortem for quantitative analysis of neurotransmitters or their enzymes. This approach has resulted in important insights into the molecular pathology of schizophrenia and neurodegenerative disorders of late life (Bird, 1980). Immunocytochemical techniques have also been applied successfully to human postmortem tissue, and demonstrate the cellular location and regional distribution of neuropeptides (Marshall & Landis, unpublished). Mass spectrophotometry may be used to survey body fluids and cellular fractions from selected brain regions for biochemical differences of potential importance for mental retardation. It is now possible to separate individual neurons from human brain tissue postmortem for precise analysis of structural proteins (Selkoe, 1980), and to isolate and sustain ribosomes and other subcellular organelles in vitro to identify and analyze the activity of short-lived cytoplasmic proteins of presumed importance for normal cellular regulation (Gilbert et al., 1981). Application of these and other technological advances to the investigation of human mental retardation can be expected to result in better understanding of etiology and pathogenesis and improved strategies for prevention and treatment in the future.

ACKNOWLEDGEMENTS

We thank Darleen Jackson and Doreen Reposa for preparation of the manuscript. Cecilia Pinto-Lord, M.D., Linda Hassinger and Robert Ferrante contributed to the illustrations. The work herein is supported in part by NIH grants 34079, 1 R01 NS 12005 and 5P30-HD 04147.

REFERENCES

Adams, R., Prod'hom, L., & Rabinowica, T. Intrauterine brain death: Neuro-axial reticular core necrosis. **Acta Neuro-pathologica**, 1977, 40, 41-49.

Bankl, H. & Jellinger, K. Zentralnervose Schaden nach fetaler Kohlenoxyvergiftung. **Beitrag Pathologisches Anatomie**, 1967, 135, 350-376.

Bird, E. A brain tissue resource center to promote research in schizophrenia. In C. Baxter & T. Melnechuck (Eds.), **Perspectives in schizophrenia research.** New York: Raven Press, 1980.

Brazier, M. & Petsche, H. **Architectonics of the Cerebral Cortex.** New York: Raven Press, 1978.

Buell, S. & Coleman, P. Quantitative evidence for selective dendritic growth in normal aging but not in senile dementia. **Brain Research**, 1981, 214, 23-41.

Cajal, S.R.-y- **Histologie du systeme nerveaux de l'homme et des vertebres**, Vol. I and II, C.I.S.C., Madrid (reprinted 1972), 1911.

Cavanagh, J. (Ed.) **The brain in unclassified mental retardation.** Baltimore: Williams and Wilkins Co., 1972.

Caviness, V. & Frost, D. Tangential organization of thalamic projections to the neocortex in the mouse. **Journal of Comparative Neurology**, 1981, **194**, 335-367.

Caviness, V. Neocortical histogenesis in normal and reeler mice: A developmental study based upon (3H)thymidine autoradiography. **Developmental Brain Research**, 4, 1982, 293-301.

Caviness, V., Evrard, P., & Lyon, G. Radial neuronal assemblies, ectopia and necrosis of the developing cortex: A case analysis. **Acta Neuropathologica**, 1978, 41, 67-72.

Caviness, V. & Rakic, P. Mechanisms of cortical development: A view from mutations in mice. **Annual Review of Neuroscience**, 1978, 1, 297-326.(b)

Caviness, V. & Williams, R. Cellular pathology of developing human cerebral cortex. In R. Katzman (Ed.), **Congenital and acquired cognitive disorders.** New York: Raven Press, 1979.

Chi, J., Dooling, E., & Gilles, F. Gyrial development of the human brain. **Annuals of Neurology**, 1977, 1, 86-93.

Christensen, E. & Melchior, J. **Cerebral palsy: A clinical and neuropathological study.** Laurenham, United Kingdom: Spastics Society Publishers, 1967.

Colonnier, M. The electron-microscopic analysis of the neuronal organization of the cerebral cortex. In F. Schmitt (Ed.), **The organization of the cerebral cortex.** Cambridge, MA: MIT Press, 1981.

Cragg, B. The density of synapses and neurons in normal, mentally defective and aging human brains. **Brain**, 1975, **98**, 81-90.

Creasy, M. & Alberman, E. Congenital malformations of the central nervous system in spontaneous abortuses. **Journal of Medical Genetics**, 1976, 13, 9-16.

Dekaban, A. Abnormalities in children exposed to x-radiation during various stages of gestation: Tentative timetable of radiation injury to the human fetus. **Journal of Nuclear Medicine**, 1968, **9**, 471.

Desmond, M. & Jacobson, A. Embryonic brain enlargement requires cerebrospinal fluid pressure. **Developmental Biology**, 1977, 57, 188-198.

Dieker, H., Edwards, R., & Zurhein, G. The lissencephaly syndrome. **Birth Defects**, 1969, 5, 53-64.

Dobbing, J. & Sands, T. Quantitative growth and development of the human brain. **Archives of Diseases of Children**, 1973, 48, 757-767.

Dooling, E. & Richardson, E. A case of adult microcephaly. **Archives of Neurology**, 1980, 37, 688-692.

Eecken, H.M. van der. **The anastemoses between the leptomeningeal arteries of the brain.** Springfield, IL: CC Thomas, 1959.

Ehlinger, G., Blakemore, C., Milner, A.D., & Wilson, J. Agenesis of the corpus callosum: A further behavioral investigation. **Brain,** 1974, **97,** 225–234.

Evrard, P., Caviness, V., & Lyon, G. The mechanism of arrest of neuronal migration in the Zellweger malformation: An hypothesis based upon cytoarchitectonic analysis. **Acta Neuropathologica,** 1978, **41,** 109–117.

Freytag, E. & Lindenberg, R. Neuropathologic findings in patients of a hospital for the mentally deficient: A survey of 359 cases. **Johns Hopkins Medical Journal,** 1967, **121,** 379–391.

Friede, R. **Developmental neuropathology.** New York: Springer, 1975.

Gilbert, J., Brown, B., Strocchi, P., Bird, E.D., & Marotta, C.A. The preparation of biologically active messenger RNA from human postmortem brain tissue. **Journal of Neurochemistry,** 1981, **36,** 976–984.

Halperin, J., Williams, R., & Kolodny, E. Microcephaly vera, progressive motor neuron disease and nigral degeneration. **Neurology** in press.

Halsey, J., Allen, N., & Chamberlan, H. The morphogenesis of hydranencephaly. **Journal of Neurological Science,** 1971, **12,** 187–217.

Huttenlocher, P. Dendritic development in neocortex of children with mental defect and infantile spasms. **Neurology,** 1974, **24,** 203–210.

Innocenti, G., Fiore, L., & Caminiti, R. Exuberant projection into the corpus callosum from the visual cortex of newborn cats. **Neuro-science Letters,** 1977, **4,** 237–242.

Jacobson, M. **Developmental neurobiology.** New York: Plenum Press, 1978.

Jones, E. Anatomy of cerebral cortex: Columnar input-output organization. In **The organization of the cerebral cortex.** Cambridge, MA: MIT Press, 1981.

Jones, E. Varieties and distribution of non-pyramidal cells in the somatic sensory cortex of the squirrel monkey. **Journal of Comparative Neurology,** 1975, **160,** 205–268.

Jones, K., Smith, D., Ulleland, C., & Streissgath, A.P. Pattern of malformation in the offspring of alcoholic mothers. **Lancet,** 1973, **1,** 1267–1271.

Kloepfer, H., Platon, R., & Hansche, W.J. Manifestations of a recessive gene for microcephaly in a population isolate. **Journal Genetik Humaine,** 1964, **13,** 52–59.

Kolliker, A. **Hanbuch der genebelehre des menchen.** Leipzig: Englemann Press, 1896.

Leck, I., Record, R., McKeown, T., & Edwards, J. The incidence of malformations in Birmingham, England, 1950–1959. **Terutalogy,** 1968, **1,** 263–280.

Lemire, R., Beckwith, J., & Warkany, J. **Anecephaly.** New York: Raven Press, 1978.

Lemire, R., Loeser, J., Leech, R., & Alvord, E. **Normal and abnormal development of the human nervous system.** New York: Harper Row, 1975.

Levine, D., Fisher, M., & Caviness, V. Porencephaly with microgyria: A pathologic study. **Acta Neuropathologica**, 1974, 29, 99–113.

Loeser, J. & Alvord, E. Agenesis of the corpus callosum. **Brain**, 1968, 91, 553–570.

Lorente de No, R. Cerebral cortex: Architecture, intracortical connections, major projections. In J. Fulton (Ed.), **Physiology of the nervous system.** New York: Oxford University Press, 1949.

Marin-Padilla, M. Prenatal and early postnatal ontogenesis of the human motor cortex: A golgi study. I. The sequential development of the cortical layers. **Brain Research**, 1970, 23, 167–183.

Marin-Padilla, M. Dual origin of the mammalian neocortex and evolution of the cortical plate. **Anatomy Embryology**, 1978, 152, 109–126.

Matthysse, S. & Williams, R. Quantitative neurohistology with the computer microscope. In C. Baxter & R. Melnechuk (Eds.), **Perspectives in schizophrenia research.** New York: Raven Press, 1980.

Molliver, M., Kostovic, I., & Van der Loos, H. The development of synapses in the cerebral cortex of the human fetus. **Brain Research**, 1973, 50, 403–407.

Moser, H. & Wolf, P. The nosology of mental retardation: Including the report of a survey of 1,378 mentally retarded individuals at the Walter E. Fernald State School. **Birth Defects**, 1971, 1, 117–134.

Mountcastle, V. The organizing principle for cerebral function: The unit module and the distributed system. In F. Schmitt (Ed.), **The neurosciences, fourth study program.** Cambridge, MA: MIT Press, 1979.

Myers, R. Brain pathology following fetal vascular occlusion: An experimental study. **Investigative Ophthalmology**, 1969, 8, 41–50.

Myers, R. & Myers, S. Use of sedative, analgesic and anesthetic drugs during labor and delivery: Bane or boon? **American Journal of Obstetrics and Gynecology**, 1979, 133, 83–104.

Myers, R., Valerio, M., Martin, D., & Nelson, K. Perinatal brain damage: Porencephaly in the cynomologous monkey. **Biological Neonate**, 1973, 22, 253–273.

Myers, R. Maternal psychological stress and fetal asphyxia: A study in the monkey. **American Journal of Obstetrics and Gynecology**, 1975, 122, 47–59.

Nauta, W. & Karten, H. A general profile of the vertebrate brain, with sidelights on the ancestry of the cerebral cortex. In F. Schmitt (Ed.), **The neurosciences: Second study program.** New York: Rochefeller University Press, 1970.

Niswander, K. & Gordon, M. **Women and their pregnancies.** Phila-
    delphia: W.B. Saunders, 1972.
Paldino, A. & Purpura, D. Quantitative analysis of the spatial
    distribution of axonal and dendritic terminals of hippocampal
    pyramidal neurons in immature human brain. **Experimental Neu-
    rology,** 1979, **64,** 604-619.
Pinto-Lord, M. & Caviness, V. Determinants of cell shape and ori-
    entation: A comparative golgi analysis of cell-axon inter-
    relationships in the developing neocortex of normal and
    reeler mice. **Journal of Comparative Neurology,** 1979, 187,
    49-70.
Purpura, D. Dendritic spine dysgenesis and mental retardation.
    Science, 1974, **186,** 1126-1128.
Purpura, D. Pathobiology of cortical neurons in metabolic and un-
    classified amentias. In R. Katzman (Ed.), **Congenital and
    acquired cognitive disorders.** New York: Raven Press, 1979.
Purpura, D., Suzuki, K., Rapin, I., & Wurzelmann, S. Dendritic
    varicosities and microtubule disarray in human cortical neu-
    rons in developmental failure. **Neuroscience Abstracts,** 1980,
    6, 339.
Rakic, P. Prenatal development of the visual system in rhesus
    monkey. **Philological Transactions Royal Society of London
    B.,** 1977, **278,** 245-260.
Rakic, P. Developmental events leading to laminar and areal or-
    ganization of neocortex. In F. Schmitt (Ed.), **The organiza-
    tion of the cerebral cortex.** Cambridge, MA: MIT Press,
    1981.
Rakic, P. & Yakovlev, P. Development of the corpus callosum and
    cavum septi in man. **Journal of Comparative Neurology,** 1968,
    132, 45-72.
Rebeiz, J., Wolf, P., & Adams, R.D. Dystrophic cortical myelino-
    genesis ("driftwood cortex"): A hitherto unrecognized form
    of developmental anomaly of the cerebrum in man. **Acta Neuro-
    pathologica,** 1968, 11, 237-252.
Richman, D., Stewart, R., & Caviness, V. Cerebral microgyria in a
    27 week fetus: An architecture and topographic analysis.
    Journal of Neuropathology and Experimental Neurology, 1974,
    33, 374-384.
Richman, D., Stewart, R., Hutchinson, J., & Caviness, V. Mechani-
    cal model of brain convolutional development. **Science,** 1975,
    189, 18-21.
Riggs, H., McGrath, J., & Schwarz, H. Malformation of the adult
    brain (albino rat) resulting from prenatal irradiation.
    Journal of Neuropathology and Experimental Neurology, 1956,
    15, 432-447.
Robain, O. & Lyon, G. Les microcephalies familiales par malfor-
    mation cerebrale. Etude Anatomoclinique. **Acta Neuropatho-
    logica,** 1972, 20, 96-109.

Selkoe, D. Altered protein composition of isolated human cortical
    neurons in Alzheimer's Disease. **Annals of Neurology**, 1980,
    8, 468-478.
Shoukimas, G. & Hinds, J. The development of cerebral cortex in
    the embryonic mouse: An electronmicroscopic serial section
    analysis. **Journal of Comparative Neurology**, 1978, **179**, 795-
    830.
Sidman, R. & Rakic, P. Neuronal migration with special reference
    to the developing human brain: A review. **Brain Research**,
    1973, **62**, 1-35.
Stewart, R., Richman, D., & Caviness, V.S. Lissencephaly and
    pachygyria: An architectonic and topographical analysis.
    Acta Neuropathologica, 1975, 31, 1-12.
Volpe, J. **Neurology of the newborn**. Philadelphia: W.B. Saunders,
    1981.
Volpe, J. & Adams, R. Cerebro-hepato-renal syndrome of Zellweger:
    An inherited disorder of neuronal migration. **Acta Neuro-
    pathologica**, 1972, **20**, 175-198.
Von Bonin, G. & Mehler, W. On the columnar arrangement of nerve
    cells in the cerebral cortex. **Brain Research**, 1971, **27**,
    1-9.
Williams, R., Ferrante, R., & Caviness, V. The cellular pathology
    of microgyria: A golgi analysis. **Acta Neuropathologica**,
    1976, 36, 269-283.
Williams, R., Hauser, S., Purpura, D.P., DeLong, G.R., & Swisher,
    C.N. Autism and mental retardation: Neuropathological
    studies performed in four retarded persons with autistic be-
    havior. **Archives of Neurology**, 1980, 37, 749-753.
Wisniewski, K., Haddad, R., Rabe, A., Dumas, R., & Shek, J. Ex-
    perimental lissencephaly in the ferret. **Journal of Neuro-
    pathology and Experimental Neurology**, 1977, 36, 638.
Yakovlev, P. Pathoarchitectonic studies of cerebral malforma-
    tions. III. Archinecephalies. **Journal of Neuropathology and
    Experimental Neurology**, 1959, 18, 22-55.

THE NEUROLOGICAL ASSESSMENT OF CHILDREN

Patricia L. Hartlage and Nicolas S. Krawiecki

Department of Pediatric Neurology
Medical College of Georgia
Athens, Georgia

Many professionals have an interest in the child with cognitive dysfunction. Each discipline has its own unique origins and traditions, uses specialized diagnostic techniques, and employs diverse treatment modalities. Cognizance of the skills of other professionals can expedite the appropriate involvement, and by knowing what they cannot do, may avoid inappropriate expectations.

Medical and psychological approaches are very different, although they are complementary to each other. Centuries of medical tradition have resulted in the physician's emphasis on the severity of a disease or disability, while clinical psychology's roots in rehabilitation have nurtured an emphasis on assessing residual abilities. This chapter, written by two physicians specializing in pediatric neurology, will address a number of issues relevant to neuropsychology: when to make a medical referral; what transpires during the typical neurological examination of a child; special ancillary diagnostic techniques; and, how the physician summarizes the clinical findings and translates them into action. The chapter concludes with several case histories that illustrate the unique contributions of the neurological physician.

MEDICAL REFERRAL

In addition to obvious health problems, there are other conditions in which a medical referral is necessary. For example, a precipitous or progressive decline in function, either physical or mental, requires prompt attention to determine if the child has a treatable disorder. Also, a child suspected of having mental retardation deserves a comprehensive medical evaluation. Even when there is no medically treatable disorder, it may be possible

Table 1. Pediatric history

<u>Family History</u>	Age and health status of siblings, parents, aunts and uncles, first cousins and grandparents.
<u>Perinatal History</u>	
Prenatal	History of previous pregnancies, diet, drugs, quality of fetal movements, health problems, and length of gestation.
Labor	Duration, difficulty, and medications used.
Delivery	Presentation (breech, or head first), forceps, caesarian delivery, annesthetics used.
Neonatal	Birth weight, jaundice or other problems needing special care. Feeding habits and activity level. Did baby go home with mother?
<u>Growth and Development</u>	
Physical growth and motor development	When did the child hold up his head, sit alone, stand, walk, and ride a tricycle?
Mental development	At what age did the child smile socially, utter his first words and phrases, feed himself, and was toilet trained? How is his school performance? Are there any behavioral problems?
<u>Nutritional History</u>	Quantity and quality.
<u>Immunization History</u>	Dates and complications.
<u>Previous Illnesses</u>	Accidents and injuries, hospitalizations, surgical procedures, specific illnesses, adverse reactions to any medical treatment, allergies.
<u>Review of Systems</u>	
Skin	Birth marks, rashes, etc.
Head	Headaches, loss of consciousness, convulsions, etc.
Eyes	Trouble seeing, crossed eyes, etc.

Nose	Discharge, bleeding, snoring, mouth breathing, etc.
Ears	Infections, earaches, trouble hearing, etc.
Throat	Infections, swallowing or speaking trouble, toothaches, etc.
Neck	Pain, lumps, stiffness, etc.
Chest	Pain, cough, wheezing, trouble breathing, etc.
Heart	Murmurs, enlargement, cyanosis, limited exercise tolerance, etc.
Gastrointestinal	Appetite, food intolerance, bowel habits, abdominal complaints, etc.
Genitourinary	Bladder habits, hernias, bedwetting, etc.
Endocrine	Problems with pubescence or menstration, etc.

to initiate interventions which could avoid recurrences of the condition. Suspicion of vision or hearing impairment is another reason for a medical evaluation. In addition, intermittent disruptions of normal functioning need to be evaluated to assess for the presence of seizures.

For any of the above conditions, the potential contribution of the physician is undisputable. Other situations also arise when a neurological evaluation might be helpful. For instance, a child with a known and previously well-evaluated handicap may benefit from a second opinion. Evaluating a child with a specific learning disability who is otherwise healthy is another reason for a neurology referral. Since all physicians operate in a problem-oriented fashion, a good guideline to use is whether in formulating an appropriate referral question the neurologist can offer something of practical use.

NEUROLOGICAL EVALUATION

MEDICAL HISTORY

Prior to examining school-age children, many neurologists obtain information which is contained in previous records and from questionnaires which are administered to parents and teachers. The actual assessment begins with direct questioning regarding the problem or symptom. In the typical medical record, this is referred to as the "chief complaint." The presenting problem is reviewed in detail to document its duration, frequency, severity, and rate of progression, as well as ameliorating and precipitating circumstances. Any associated symptoms are also recorded.

Next, the physician conducts a systematic review of the health history. The specific areas covered are presented in Table 1. Because of its obvious importance, a pediatric neurologist directs a considerable amount of the questioning to events surrounding the perinatal period and developmental history. In practice, more time is expended gathering historical data than in the examination of the child, since this has been proven to be the most valuable part of the physician's assessment.

THE PHYSICAL EXAMINATION

The pediatric neurologist conducts a general physical examination of the patient before proceeding to an examination of nervous system functioning. During the physical examination, findings may emerge which are very important to understanding how the nervous system is working. For example, hemiplegia, which has a very early onset in life, may cause the affected arm and leg to grow less well than the opposite limbs. This growth asymmetry may persist, even though strength returns to the once affected limbs. Congenital abnormalities in other organs can also be associated with cerebral dysfunction. Among the most classic syndromes affecting neurological development are those resulting from chromosomal disturbances.

The value of a general physical examination is illustrated in the fact that much importance is attached to examining a child's skin. Both the skin and the central nervous system originate embryologically from the ectoderm. It is not surprising, therefore, that developmental defects might be reflected in both tissues. A number of neurocutaneous syndromes exist in which characteristic birth marks often are the first clue that a disorder exists which may profoundly affect brain function. White "ash leaf" spots are present from birth in children with tuberous sclerosis; a syndrome that is associated with a high incidence of epilepsy and mental retardation. Light brown "cafe au lait" spots are the hallmarks of neurofibromatosis. This is another disorder in which there is an increased risk for neurological dysfunction and tumors of the nervous system. A "port wine" birth mark on the face is often associated with a similar birthmark on the brain, resulting in the Sturge-Weber syndrome. Tuberous sclerosis and neurofibromatosis are autosomal dominant hereditary disorders, but Sturge-Weber syndrome is not hereditary. In the disorder resulting from chromosome errors, the skin abnormalities are often revealed in the dermatoglyphic pattern; that is, finger prints and creases of the palms and soles. Skin pigmentation may be altered by other diseases of neurological importance. For example, children with phenylketonuria have lighter pigmentation. Excessive pigmentation is seen in adrenocortical leukodystrophy, a hereditary degenerative disease of the adrenal gland and nervous system. The appearance of the skin, hair, and teeth, as well as body growth, show characteristic changes due to hypothyroidism in children. Space limitations do not allow for a more detailed discussion of the entire general physical examination, but the above discussion illustrates the rationalized importance of the pediatric neurologist.

If not recorded as part of the general physical examination, careful note is first made of the child's general appearance and behavior. The younger the child, the more the findings of the neurological examination are influenced by the behavioral state of the patient. The child who is frightened, sleepy, hungry, or cold could potentially yield findings that are not a valid reflection of neurological status.

Regardless of the age of the patient, the neurologist records the findings of his examination in the following standard format: (1) **Mental (or developmental) status**; (2) **Cranial nerve function**; (3) **Motor function**; and, (4) **Sensory function**.

Infant examination. This evaluation begins with the patient in the mother's lap where the neurologist can innocuously assess the infant's activity level, alertness, spontaneous movements, vocalizations and social interactions. Vision and hearing, as well as movements of the eyes, face, head, neck and upper and lower extremities can all be assessed without having to touch the child. Gradually, the head is palpated, the limbs are moved to assess tone, and assessments are made of muscle strength reflexes, and response to tactile stimuli. The heart, lungs and cranium are listened to with a stethoscope.

Next, the child is undressed and placed on a table so that observations of motor skills and developmental reflexes can be made. Certain reflexes are characteristic of particular age levels and either their absence or their persistence beyond the normal age may indicate brain problems. Asymmetries in these reflexes raise suspicion of lateralized cerebral dysfunction. In Table 2, three examples of developmental reflexes are presented.

Palpation of the abdomen and examination of the spine, skin and genitalia are next conducted. Then an effort is made to visualize the child's retina and optic discs with an ophthalmoscope while the child is either on the table or on the mother's lap. Toward the end of the evaluation, when cooperation is of less vital importance, the ears and throat are examined. Throughout the examination, the child's gross and fine motor development, and receptive and expressive language and social skills are continuously being evaluated and compared to parental reports of the developmental skills.

Table 2. Examples of developmental reflexes

Reflexes	Description	Time Present
Moro	Hold child supine. Allow head to fall backwards about 30°.	Prominent from birth to 2 months
	Arms fling up and outwards, hands open. Then arms come in.	Vestiges present 6 months
Tonic neck response	Turn head to the side in supine position.	Birth to 6 months
	Arm and leg extend on side to which head is turned, opposite limbs flex.	Most prominent at 2 months
Landau	In ventral suspension flexion of the head is followed by flexion of the legs or the trunk	8-24 months

The foregoing describes the standard examination given to all infants. In practice, if the history suggests a specific problem area, or if in the course of observing and examining the baby some problem is noted, the physicians will explore the possibility of a localized anatomic lesion. For example, if a six-month-old child is developmentally too young to have established a preference, but nonetheless is "definitely left handed," the hypothesis could be advanced that the child may have either a left hemisphere lesion or right arm nerve damage. Hence, left hemisphere functions would be specifically emphasized during the course of the examination. Information concerning the child's posture, movement, and tone, as well as reflexes of the right side of the face, right arm and leg, awareness of stimulation of the right side of the body, and awareness of objects in the right visual field, is obtained. If these functions are unimpaired, the possibility of damage to the nerve supplying the right arm is then assessed by inspection of the arm for muscle atrophy of fasciculations (small twitchings) along with an evaluation of individual muscles of the arm and individual sensory dermatomes.

Examination of the older child. The history-taking procedure for older children is identical to that for infants and young children. However, there is an additional source of information which is of utmost importance; namely, the child's school performance and behavior in the classroom. Ideally, this information should be obtained and reviewed prior to the child's visit to the clinic. If available, the results of psychological evaluations can also provide useful information to the pediatric neurologist, particularly if it is suspected that academic underachievement is a result of a disturbance of higher cerebral function.

The physical examination assesses for the presence of disease that also affects the central nervous system. The case reports at the end of this chapter are good illustrations of several disorders in which this is commonly seen. The neurological examination is generally performed in an orderly fashion. A typical sequence involves the examination of cranial nerves, motor function, reflexes, and sensory capacities.

Mental status. The mental status examination assesses higher cerebral functions. This portion of the examination is by no means a psychological or neuropsychological assessment but it, nonetheless, enables the physician to formulate some judgments regarding overall functioning. Awareness and interest in the surroundings indicates how alert the child is. Attention to the environment is inferred by the extent to which the child plays with toys, reads books, acts drowsy, or falls asleep if left to himself. Assessing attention is a very difficult task and the findings are not necessarily indicative of how the child behaves at home or in school. However, having the child perform certain tasks such as visual and verbal sequencing tests, copying simple drawings, and recalling a short story, can be very informative in regard to attention capacities.

Speech and language are informally assessed during verbal exchanges with the child. From such interaction, an understanding of the child's fluency, articulation, vocabulary and syntax can be obtained. Comprehension is tested by asking the patient to perform a few simple tasks. If necessary, more comprehensive and standardized testing can be conducted by a speech and language pathologist.

Reading is tested by presenting age-appropriate reading material. Silent reading, as well as reading aloud, are assessed. Comprehension of the material questioned is also checked. Short-term memory can be tested, as well, by asking the patient to recall the contents of a paragraph. By testing recall again after 45 minutes, it is possible to get some measure of long-term or delayed memory. Other measures include penmanship, writing under dictation and writing from a model. In addition, the child's ability to do arithmetic calculations is evaluated.

The mental status examination is not as standardized as the other portions of the neurological examination. When standardized scores are required, the neurologist will refer to an occupational therapist or neuropsychologist for assessment. However, the information can often detect impairments of the high cerebral functions through the above procedures that are clarified and elaborated upon with more formal standardized testing.

Cranial nerve examination. This procedure follows the traditional neurological format:

Cranial nerve I (olfactory): This is examined by testing the patient's sense of smell. In pediatric neurology, anosmia, or absence of smell, is very rarely observed.

Cranial nerve II (optic): This nerve pathway is directly responsible for vision. Visual acuity is tested. Visual fields are generally examined by a confrontation method in which the patient's visual fields are compared to the examiner's. In addition, the optic nerve and the retina are visualized during the fundoscopic examination, using a hand-held ophthalmoscope.

Cranial nerve III (oculomotor), IV (trochlear), and VI (abducens): These nerves are tested by examining ocular movements and noting the presence of eye deviation. Pupillary reactions to light and accommodation and position of the eye lids are checked.

Cranial nerve V (trigeminal): This nerve is tested by assessing facial sensation and the muscles of mastication.

Cranial nerve VII (facial): This nerve, controlling the muscles of facial expression and taste in part of the tongue, is tested accordingly.

Cranial nerve VIII (acoustic): This nerve is tested by assessing hearing capacity. If a deficit is suspected, a referral should be made for a complete audiological evaluation. Balance is partially controlled by the vestibular component of the cranial nerve.

Cranial nerve IX (glossopharyngeal) and X (vagus): These nerves are difficult to test clinically. Routinely, the gag reflex is elicited, and the movements of the soft palate are observed. The quality of the patient's voice can also indicate if the nerves are not functioning normally.

Cranial nerve XI (spinal accessory): This nerve innervates the muscles of the neck and shoulders. It is tested by assessing the strength of the neck muscles which turn the head and the ability of the patient to shrug his or her shoulders.

Cranial nerve XII (hypoglossal): This nerve innervates the muscles of the tongue and is tested by assessing tongue movements.

Motor examination. This component of the neurological examination assesses the muscles, nerves to the muscles, motor pathways in the spinal cord, the voluntary motor control centers in the cerebral cortex, and the complex components of the involuntary motor centers such as the basal ganglia and cerebellum. Muscles are inspected for appearance at rest, for tone (the resistance to passive movements of the joints), and for strength.

Specific motor activities are observed during standing posture, walking, running and arising from a sitting position on the floor. The child is also asked to stand and hop on each leg, to walk on their heels, on their toes and finally with one foot in front of the other. The capacity of the patient to perform rapid alternating movements is observed along with the child's accuracy in pointing at a target. Equilibrium is also tested as part of the motor examination. Abnormalities found on the motor examination have highly localizing value, and only a modicum of patient cooperation is needed for the neurologist to conduct a comprehensive survey of the essential elements of the motor system.

Reflexes. The primitive reflexes found in the infant are normally no longer present in the older child. The muscle stretch reflexes are elicited by tapping the tendons of the muscles. These reflexes are tested for the biceps, triceps, brachioradialis for the upper extremities, and the quadriceps and achilles for the lower extremities. The superficial reflexes commonly elicited are the abdominal, and in males, the cremasteric reflexes. Some reflexes, such as an extensor response to stimulation of the plantar surface of the foot, also called the Babinski sign, are pathognomonic of motor dysfunction in the central nervous system.

Sensory examination. This is probably the most difficult part of the neurological examination. By definition, it is a subjective examination, since the patient is asked to analyze and respond to a stimulus. It requires maximum cooperation, and because of this prerequisite, it is often difficult to conduct in children, especially those with severe neurological dysfunction.

Various types of sensation are tested. These include touch, pain, vibratory sense, and position sense. The sensory experiences are all transmitted to the brain via different anatomical pathways which make this aspect of the examination very useful for a specific lesion. Simultaneous bilateral stimulation is conducted as a quick assessment of parietal lobe function. Stereognosis

Table 3.   Commonly employed neurodiagnostic tests

Neuroradiological Tests

Plain Skull Films: Bony structures of the skull are visualized.
It is often helpful in the evaluation of severe head injury.
It can reveal calcified areas within the brain in cases of
prenatal infection, neurocutaneous disease, and in some types
of slow growing tumors.   When standard X-ray equipment was
all that was available, a clearer delineation of intracranial
structures was possible only by using certain contrast media
(such as air that is introduced by lumbar puncture (penumo-
encephalograph), radio-opaque dyes that are injected into
blood vessels (angiography), or by lumbar puncture around the
spinal cord (myelography).

Computerized Tomograms (CT scan):   Intracranial structures, as well
as bones, are visualized.   The CT scan can delineate abnormal
fluid collections (e.g., hydrocephalus or subdural hematomas),
aneurysms, congenital malformations, focal areas of atrophy,
and calcifications.

Neurophysiological Tests

Electroencephalogram (EEG):   The EEG records the electrical rhythms
of the brain.   This technique is an important adjunct in the
diagnosis of epilepsy, particularly if a seizure can be recorded.

Electromyography (EMG):   The EMG records the electrical activity in
muscles.   It is used to detect and differentiate between diseases affecting the motor nerve cells of the spinal cord, the
peripheral nerves, the neuromuscular junction and the muscle
itself.

Nerve Conduction Velocities: This procedure is usually performed in
conjunction with the EMG.   Conduction velocities are determined
by measuring the responses to electric stimulation of the peripheral nerves.   Both motor and sensory nerves can be evaluated
by this method.

Computer Averaged Evoked Responses: The averaged electrical response of the brain to a series of auditory, visual or somato-
sensory stimuli are recorded.   The best established use in
clinical practice is for the quantification of hearing loss
by measuring the brain stem auditory evoked response.

Biopsy of a Body Tissue or Fluid

Lumbar Puncture and Spinal Fluid Examination: This procedure is
    primarily used in the diagnosis of infectious diseases. The
    spinal fluid can, in addition, reflect a variety of disease
    processes in the nervous system.

Samples of blood, urine, skin and muscle can often be used to
    diagnosis metabolic and degenerative diseases that affect the
    central nervous system, although the sophistication of the
    tests may require shipping the tissue to specially equipped
    laboratories.

(ability to recognize objects by feeling their shape and texture
with the eyes closed) and graphesthesia (ability to recognize
drawing done on the palm of the hands with the eyes closed) are
also routinely conducted.

At the conclusion of the traditional neurological examination, the physician should be able to answer three specific questions: (1) Is there a neurological dysfunction? (2) Where in the
brain is the dysfunction? And, (3) What is the nature of the dysfunction?   As a rule, laboratory tests and other special procedures should not be used to arrive at the answers to these questions, but rather to confirm or disconfirm a diagnostic impression
which is based on the history, physical examination and neurological examination.   Some commonly employed tests are described in
Table 3.

CASE HISTORIES

The following are case histories illustrating some childhood
behavior problems where the neurologist has been able to make a
contribution.

A BOY WITH PECULIAR MANNERISMS

Paul, age four and a half, was brought to the emergency room
late one evening by his mother, a nurse at the same hospital.
"He's been acting crazy all day. He can't sit still, and I just
wanted to be sure there was nothing physically wrong." Paul
appeared to be in excellent health. At first, the emergency room
physician was puzzled since his examination revealed no abnormalities. Then Paul suddenly stood up, jumped, tossed his head and
shivered his entire body. This same sequence was repeated every
few minutes, although the youngster could attend and converse normally during these gyrations. A mild sedative was prescribed and

an appointment with a child psychiatrist was suggested. The sedative was effective and Paul slept peacefully that night. However, the same sequence occurred the next day. Paul did not seem particularly upset by these disturbances and went about his usual routine, although it was interrupted by the recurrent unusual motor events. The mother, suspecting that her son might have some form of epilepsy, consulted a psychiatrically trained neurologist.

When the consultation was arranged several days later, the symptoms had subsided considerably, although Paul was still tossing his head at intervals and occasionally made peculiar noises. The mother told the neurologist that Paul was a healthy youngster who had reached both motor and verbal milestones sooner than her friends' children. He had been seen by an ophthalmologist at age two because of eye blinking, but at that time no problems were found. In addition, he had been under the care of an allergist for approximately a year for frequent spells of sniffing and coughing which did not respond very well to treatment.

The neurologist suspected Tourette's Syndrome, an involuntary movement disorder that features motor and verbal tics which wax and wane in both character and severity. The verbal tics often take the form of grunting, barking, screaming or shouting obscenities. The onset of the symptoms is between two and thirteen years of age. A family history of this disorder is often present. The tics or habit spasms can be voluntarily suppressed, at times for a moment or two and at other times for hours. Intellect is not impaired. The finding that there was suppression of Paul's syndrome after the administration of small doses of haloperidol strengthened the diagnosis of Tourette's Syndrome. This drug is capable of blocking dopamine receptors in the extrapyramidal or involuntary motor system, suggesting that the disorder stems from a hypersensitivity to the dopamine neurotransmitter.

Tourette's Syndrome and other disorders of involuntary movement are often mistaken for psychological problems. Typically, however, psychological testing does not reveal either cognitive or emotional problems. Often, many years elapse before the problem is correctly diagnosed. While the causes are physical, the treatment must include both medication and supportive counseling, since the psychosocial impact of suffering from this disorder is usually more disabling than the actual symptoms.

AN UNUSUAL LOOKING FIRST GRADER

Because John had not been able to keep pace with his classmates, it was recommended that he repeat the first grade. Group testing at the end of the school year revealed that he was performing at the early first grade level. The teacher individually administered the Peabody Picture Vocabulary Test, yielding an IQ equivalent of 115. His drawing of a human figure, scored by the Goodenough norms, indicated an IQ equivalent of 85. Because of the discrepancy in scores, the teacher suggested a medical examination in order to rule out the possibility of vision or hearing problems. She did not specifically voice a concern about the fact that John's physical appearance was unusual.

The physician's diagnosis was formed when John entered the room with his older-than-average mother. His facial features, body habits, and the appearance of his hands and feet were characteristic of children with Down's Syndrome. Because John was socially poised and well-spoken, skills that were probably acquired in an especially stimulating and verbal home environment, and was slightly taller and thinner than average, he did not appear to the teacher like the few other Down's children she had seen. Formal psychometric assessment that year with the Stanford-Binet, and three years later with the Weschler Intelligence Scale for Children-Revised yielded IQs in the high 50's range. Chromosome analysis confirmed the presence of an extra number 21 chromosome. John was transferred to a class for the educable mentally retarded for his second year.

Particular types of physical findings may have useful diagnostic and prognostic value. Chromosome errors are only one example. Identification of syndromes resulting from the fetal exposure to alcohol and certain drugs may help prevent similar problems in subsequent offspring. Even the recognition of syndromes which are non-genetic and nontreatable may also be helpful in planning and setting reasonable parental expectations. For instance, the Cornelia de Lange Syndrome characterized by dwarfism, hirsutism and short mid-face is usually associated with severe mental impairment, while the Williams "elfin facies" Syndrome is usually predictive of much milder mental impairment. Specific craniofacial abnormalities are sometimes associated with brain malformations and dysfunctions. Extremely close-set eyes are usually associated with an incomplete separation of the cerebral hemispheres and severe retardation. Yet, children with extremely wide set eyes typically have normal brains. An extremely wide head carries a risk for retardation, while an extremely large head carries virtually no risk.

A LANGUAGE-DELAYED PRESCHOOLER

Denise was first seen at age three. She was a petite youngster who had attained normal motor milestones. However, she did not use single words until 18 months of age and was still speaking in phrases at the time of the consultation. The pregnancy and delivery were uncomplicated. At birth, Denise weighed 8 pounds. She had been in good health except for three mysterious illnesses that began with what appeared to be a relatively mild infection of the upper respiratory tract and extreme lethargy that lasted several days. Her eating habits were described as peculiar in that she exhibited a preference for sweets and starchy vegetables along with a marked dislike for meat.

Upon physical examination, she was alert and obtained scores in the third percentile for height, weight, and head size. She was slightly immature in her coordination and very immature in her language skills. Her hair was short and had been either rubbed or broken off in patches.

The characteristics that she displayed, including the food preferences, hair loss, and periods of lethargy, suggested a metabolic or nutritional disorder. An amino acid chromatogram performed on a random urine specimen disclosed the excretion of large amounts of arginino-succinic acid, an intermediary compound that is involved in the conversion of ammonia to urea in protein metabolism. An enzyme assay performed on her red blood cells confirmed the absence of the enzyme arginino-succininase. Consequently, a low protein diet was instituted that was supplemented with arginine. Within several months, an improvement in body and hair growth was apparent. Despite this regimen, however, she was still functioning in only the high educable range of mental retardation ten years later.

After the identification of phenylketonuria, the first treatable inborn error of metabolism that causes mental retardation, a number of other defects that are responsive to early dietary interventions have been discovered. Most states presently have compulsory screening programs to test newborns for the most common defects. Because it is not possible to screen for all types of defects, in cases where there is an inexplicably slowly developing youngster, searching for a metabolic disturbance is warranted.

LANGUAGE DISTURBANCE AFTER THE ONSET OF SEIZURES IN AN OLDER CHILD

Kevin had always been a highly verbal youngster. He was the narrator for the Christmas play in first grade. An excellent student, he was reading at the third grade level in the middle of the first grade, and fifth grade level in the middle of the second grade.

Kevin had two seizures, one in the spring of first grade, and one in the fall of second grade. In the spring of second grade, he began to have trouble following verbal directions, and his teacher and parents noticed he was beginning to lip read. The school audiologist reported that Kevin had a normal pure tone audiogram. His speech audiogram was inconsistent and "compatible with malingering."

Despite these problems, Kevin was evaluated for placement in a gifted program at the beginning of third grade. An IQ score of 125 was obtained. On the Peabody Individual Achievement Test, he was achieving at the following grade levels: Mathematics, 4.4 grade level; Reading Recognition, 5.0 grade level; and, Reading Comprehension, 6.5 grade level.

Kevin was first seen by a pediatric neurologist at about this time because of continued deterioration in his speech. The examination was normal, except that on one occasion he exhibited what appeared to be a pure word deafness, and on another occasion a marked receptive and expressive dysphasia. The EEG revealed right temporal or bitemporal spike discharges. The CT scan showed no structural lesion. Treatment was initiated with Dilantin (phenytoin) and the dose was increased until signs of toxicity were experienced. Despite this regimen no obvious improvements were noted. When the dose was slightly decreased, Kevin had a generalized seizure and stopped talking entirely for two weeks. Tegretol (carbamazepine) was then introduced. When high therapeutic blood levels were achieved, his expressive language improved and he seemed to engage in less lip reading. Attempts to reduce his Tegretol dosage were followed by temporary language deterioration. Increasing the dosage beyond the usual recommended level resulted in some mild clumsiness; however, a gradual improvement in both receptive and expressive language, with coincidental gradual improvement of his EEG, also occurred. After one year on this program, the EEG and language abilities returned to normal.

REFERENCES

A series of monographs, **Clinics in Developmental Medicine**, produced by Spastics International Medical Publications, are the most widely regarded descriptions of the neurological examination of infants and children. These classic monographs, published in Philadelphia by J.B. Lippincott Co., are:

Andre'e-Thomas, S., Chesni, Y., & Saint-Anne Dargassies, S. **The neurological examination of the infant.** (1960)

Brazelton, T.B. **Neonatal behavioral assessment scale.** (1973)

Dubowitz, L., & Dubowitz, V. **The neurological assessment of the preterm and full-term newborn infant.** (1981)

Paine, R.S., & Opp'e, T.E. **Neurological examination of children.** (1966)

Prechtl, H.F.R. **The neurological examination of the full-term infant.** 2nd Edition (1977)

QUANTITATIVE APPROACHES TO THE NEUROPSYCHOLOGICAL ASSESSMENT OF CHILDREN

Byron P. Rourke

Department of Psychiatry
University of Windsor
Windsor, Ontario

and

Kenneth M. Adams

Department of Psychiatry
Henry Ford Hospital
Detroit, Michigan

It would seem virtually axiomatic that the aim of psychological inquiry as it relates to the assessment of children is to produce a system for this purpose that is objective and consensually validatable. Whether such a system need be quantitative is a moot point. Certainly, there are many who would argue that a qualitative approach to assessment can be at least as objective and as open to consensual validation as are any quantitative approaches (e.g., Luria & Majovski, 1977).

Be that as it may, this chapter was not designed to compare the relative merits of the quantitative versus qualitative approaches to neuropsychological assessment of children. Rather, its aims are as follows: (a) to describe and explicate a number of salient features of the quantitative approach, and to make some statements regarding their relative merits and shortcomings; and, (b) to elucidate some ways in which quantitative assessment data can be analyzed with maximal benefits by employing a planned program of multivariate statistical investigative techniques.

A further limitation with respect to the matters discussed in this chapter is that we have confined ourselves to an examination of quantitative methods of assessment that are standardized and

which attempt to exploit the so-called "battery" approach to
assessment. Although it would certainly seem possible that indi-
vidualized forms of quantitative assessment that are designed specifically for a particular child would be amenable to objective
and validatable analysis, these particular modi operandi are very
difficult to structure within the terms of reference of actuarial
approaches to assessment -- a major focus of this chapter. Thus,
what we propose to do is to examine distinctive aspects of quantitative approaches to the neuropsychological assessment of children
that are standardized and uniform (in the sense that all tests are
given to all children in the same manner regardless of the nature
of their presenting neuropsychological problem) and to examine the
prospects for the application of actuarial procedures for the
analysis of such quantitative data.

ESSENTIAL ASPECTS OF THE NEUROPSYCHOLOGICAL ASSESSMENT BATTERY

The principal criteria against which the adequacy of a neuropsychological assessment produced for children must be judged are
(a) reliability, (b) validity, and (c) coverage.

Reliability. The specific dimensions of reliability that are
most important relate to inter-rater reliability and test-retest
reliability. It is obvious that attempts to create standardized
assessment procedures for children have as their aim the generating of tests that have very high inter-rater or inter-examiner
reliabilities. Certainly, reliability coefficients that fall
below .90 would be completely unacceptable for this purpose.
Indeed, most neuropsychologists would aim for reliabilities that
fall much closer to 1.00 than to .90. The other type of reliability that is very important in this connection, test-retest reliability, need not generate reliability coefficients as high as
those necessary for inter-rater reliabilities. However, testing
procedures that generate reliability coefficients below .85 for
test-retest periods of up to one week would be quite unacceptable
for most purposes. (Clear exceptions to this rule are reliabilities obtained on test-retest procedures administered to children
who are in the throes of rapidly deteriorating or rapidly improving neuropsychological status.)

Another type of reliability, that is, internal consistency,
is of obvious importance for procedures that require items of
equal difficulty and which do not have timed requirements. Tests
of selective and sustained attention and vigilance are examples of
measures where internal consistency can be of particular importance. However, in general, the principal dimensions of reliability that are germane to the neuropsychological assessment of children are inter-rater and test-retest types of reliability.

Validity. The principal focus of concern with respect to the validity of neuropsychological measures is the extent to which these measures are valid from a concurrent and predictive standpoint. For example, there are many who would maintain that the major purpose of a neuropsychological assessment is to determine the current structural and functional integrity of brain systems through the use of neuropsychological assessment procedures. However, this constitutes only one type of concurrent validity, albeit a rather important one. Concurrent validity coefficients in the .60s are usually considered to be the lower-bound levels of acceptance for a neuropsychological procedure that is designed for clinical use. However, most would maintain that considerably more than 50 percent of the variance should be accounted for and, hence, would suggest that concurrent validity coefficients should be in the .70s or even the .80s before being considered useful for most neuropsychological assessment purposes.

Although not as often focused upon, the question of predictive validity should be of considerable concern to the child neuropsychologist. The reasons for this are fairly straightforward. First, it is often the case that the child neuropsychologist is asked to make predictions on the basis of neuropsychological assessment procedures regarding how important it would be to institute habilitational and rehabilitational procedures for a given child. Without some knowledge of the likely course of a given condition, it would be impossible to state with any degree of confidence whether therapeutic intervention is necessary. Secondly, there are many neuropsychological conditions which afflict children that require close physiological and behavioral monitoring. For example, a particular type of seizure disorder (e.g., psychomotor epilepsy) may eventuate in rather more difficult environmental interactions for an adolescent than would some other types of seizure disorder (e.g., petit mal seizures). Alerting parents and other caretakers to these eventualities, as well as to the necessity for an ongoing interaction between assessment and intervention, falls within the rubric of predictive validity. Although it is very often the case that such predictions are based on data gathered outside of the quantitative neuropsychological assessment, it is also likely that a thoroughgoing analysis of the latter can be quite instructive with respect to the rather long-range problems to which the child, and later the adolescent and adult, may be subject.

A very good example of the double considerations of concurrent and predictive validity as these apply to the neuropsychological aspects of reading disabilities is the recent investigation of Fletcher and Satz (1980). In this study, these investigators demonstrated how the same measurements can be used for both the determination of current reading status and for the prediction of eventual reading status. This type of co-determination should be the focus of procedures used to evaluate neuropsychological assessment methods.

Coverage. Apart from the psychometric properties of reliability and validity, the most important consideration and criterion of evaluation for neuropsychological assessment procedures is the extent to which the measures obtained with any particular procedure do "justice" to the abilities known to be subserved by the cerebral hemispheres, and which are known to be disturbed when the systems within the brain are dysfunctional and/or damaged. Reitan (1966) is the neuropsychologist most closely associated with the accentuation of the importance of this particular dimension of assessment. He has consistently pointed to the absolute necessity of obtaining an adequate sampling of the brain's principal systems if reasonable assertions are to emerge from neuropsychological assessments.

It should be noted that this is particularly important within the present context because procedures that purport to be amenable to programmatic, actuarial modes of interpretation are radically dependent upon the completeness of the data that are submitted to any particular actuarial algorithm. The systematic limitation of data utilized within these types of data manipulation and judgment-generating techniques would be expected to have a profound impact upon the concurrent and predictive validity of the statements generated by them. However, even apart from considerations germane to actuarial purposes, it would seem obvious that the tests and measures employed in any neuropsychological battery should "cover" the content and styles of information analysis, organization, and synthesis, together with input, output, and coordination dimensions, so as to provide a reasonably complete catalogue of the behaviors that can be impaired when the brain of the child is functioning in an abnormal fashion.

In order to illustrate this point more clearly, a particular neuropsychological battery designed for use with children will be discussed. The tests used in this battery are displayed in Table 1. These tests are categorized in terms of a system suggested by Reitan (1974). However, it should be borne in mind that not all tests fall neatly within these categories and that there is considerable overlap between them. Indeed, given the fact that the brain's systems are, in large measures, interdependent, it should come as no surprise that this would have to be the case.

There are several aspects of this neuropsychological test battery that should be commented upon in connection with the issue of coverage. For example, it should be noted that the tests and measures in this battery include measures of sensory-perceptual, motor and psychomotor, psycholinguistic, and concept-formation and problem solving abilities. In addition, within each of these

Table 1. Tests Included in Neuropsychological Test Battery

TACTILE-PERCEPTUAL

    Reitan-Klove Tactile-Perceptual and Tactile Form Recognition
       Tests

       Tactile Imperception and Suppression
       Finger Agnosia
       Fingertip Number-Writing Recognition (older)
       Fingertip Symbol-Writing Recognition (FSWR)(Younger)
       Coin Recognition (Older)
       Tactile-Form Recognition (Younger)

VISUAL-PERCEPTION

    Reitan-Klove Visual Perceptual Tests
    Target Test
    Constructional Dyspraxia Items, Halstead-Wepman Aphasia
       Screening Test

    WISC Picture Completion, Picture Arrangement, Block Design,
       Object Assembly Subtests

    Trail Making Test for Children, Part A (Older)
    Color Form Test (Younger)
    Progressive Figures Test (Younger)
    Individual Performances Tests (Younger)

       Matching Figures
       Star Drawing
       Matching Vs
       Concentric Squares Drawing

AUDITORY-PERCEPTUAL AND LANGUAGE-RELATED

    Reitan-Klove Auditory-Perceptual Test
    Seashore Rhythm Test
    Speech-Sounds Perception Test
    Auditory Closure Test (Kass, 1964)
    Sentence Memory Test (Benton, 1965)
    Verbal Fluency Test
    Peabody Picture Vocabulary Test (Dunn, 1965)
    Aphasoid Items, Aphasia Screening Test

    WISC Information, Comprehension, Similarities,
       Vocabularly, Digit Span Subtests

(continued overleaf)

PROBLEM SOLVING, CONCEPT FORMATION, REASONING

Halstead Category Test
WISC Arithmetic Subtest
Children's Word Finding Test (Pajurkova, Orr, Rourke,
    & Finlayson, 1976)
Matching Pictures Test (Younger)

MOTOR AND PSYCHOMOTOR

Reitan–Klove Lateral Dominance Examination
Dynamometer
Finger Tapping Test
Foot Tapping Test
Klove–Matthews Motor Steadiness Battery

Maze Coordination Test
Static Steadiness
Grooved Pegboard Test

OTHER

Underlining Test (Doehring, 1968; Rourke & Orr, 1977)
WISC Coding Subtest
Tactual Performance Test
Trail Making Test for Children, Part B (Older)

---

fairly broad categories, an attempt has been made to include rather homogeneous tests, as well as those that are heterogenous with respect to the abilities that are presumably necessary for their successful handling. Related to this are the inclusion of measures that vary along the "easy-difficult" and "simple-complex" dimensions.

An example of the application of these principles can be gleaned from a consideration of the tests listed within the Motor and Psychomotor category. In this instance, rather simple motor skills, such as strength of grip and tapping speed, are examined, followed by somewhat more complex psychomotor skills, such as static and kinetic steadiness, which in turn are followed by the testing of the fairly complex dimensions of fine eye-hand coordination under speeded conditions. Within this category, it is fairly easy to see the "simple-complex" dimension. What may not be so obvious is the "easy-difficult" dimension. In fact, the very definitions of "easy" and "difficult" change as a function of the particular neuropathological condition from which the child may be suffering. For example, a child who has a medulloblastoma within the cerebellum would be expected to have particular difficulty with the Maze test of kinetic tremor, whereas he/she might have little or no difficulty with the Holes test of static tremor. This would stand in marked contrast to a child with a basal ganglia lesion that hampered both kinetic and static steadiness skills, and to one with a lateralized lesion of the motor strip where all motor skills (simple and complex) on only one side of the body are impaired.

Also included in this neuropsychological test battery are tests that require inter-sensory integration, novel problem-solving, and higher-order concept-formation and strategy-generating capacities. An example of a test that requires all of these elements for its successful completion is the Tactual Performance Test (Reitan & Davison, 1974). On this test, the child is required to integrate simple and complex stimuli delivered through the tactile mode with aspects of kinesthetic feedback and visual imagery; this must be done within a situation that requires him/her to be blindfolded and to carry out a problem-solving task under conditions that are anything but common for the vast majority of children; he/she must also be able to generate an adequate problem-solving strategy, change that strategy in the light of new information, and carry out a consistent mode of approach once an effective plan is generated.

One important reason for the inclusion of tests such as this is that measures of adaptive abilities that require the capacity to deal with novelty tend to be far more sensitive to the effects of brain dysfunction than do tasks of a more rote or programmatic nature (Reitan, 1966). Of course, this is not always the case, and it is for this reason that a number of measures of highly overlearned skills are also included in this battery of tests. In addition, there is accumulating empirical evidence and an emerging theoretical perspective that suggests that systematic comparisons of the individual's characteristic manner of dealing with novel vs. rote or routinized information may have significance with respect to the relative differential integrity of the two cerebral hemispheres (Goldberg & Costa, 1981; Rourke, 1982a). In order to determine the significance of this dimension in the individual case, it should be clear that the actuarial comparison of various aspects of the novelty-rote dichotomy could be of considerable assistance. Indeed, virtually every aspect of the dimensions tapped by this battery and others like it (including, for example, speeded vs. power tests, measures involving sensory-perceptual abilities within a framework of little or no vs. a great deal of psychomotor coordination) can be handled much more systematically, with greater precision, and with a higher likelihood of replication with the decision making aided by programmatic actuarial algorithms.

CLINICAL INTERPRETATIVE STRATEGIES AND THE QUANTITATIVE APPROACH TO NEUROPSYCHOLOGICAL ASSESSMENT

In-depth examinations of the manner in which clinical inter-pretative strategies have been employed in conjunction with the type of neuropsychological test battery described in this chapter have been examined elsewhere (Rourke, 1975, 1976, 1978, 1981, 1982b; Rourke, Bakker, Fisk, & Strang, 1983). Our purpose here is simply to explain how the quantitative/actuarial approach can be used to good advantage by the clinician who is inclined to employ these interpretative strategies. To that end, brief remarks regarding the salience of quantitative data for these strategies are offered.

Level of performance. Clinical interpretation of test data from a level of performance perspective has been a traditional mainstay within the clinical psychologist's arsenal of interpre-tative techniques. With adults, the brain damage vs. no brain damage diagnostic decision has long been couched within this frame of reference. However, few serious clinical neuropsychologists are any longer interested in the application of this interpreta-tive strategy in order to answer this particular question. Some of the reasons for this are as follows: (1) there are relatively few clinical advantages to making this decision correctly; (2) there are very obvious shortcomings that inhere within an approach to the analysis of performance that does not take into consideration the large number of potentially limiting psychosocial and psycho-physiological conditions other than brain damage that can affect performance on neuropsychological tests in an adverse fashion; and, (3) the decision, once made, has little or no relevance for rehabilitation.

However, especially with children (and with oldsters), the systematic comparisons of the individual's performances with developmental norms can yield an enormous amount of valuable information. This being the case, it goes almost without saying that programmatic comparisons of a child's performance on a battery of neuropsychological tests with developmentally appro-priate norms for these tests would be highly desirable. This takes on added significance when we come to consider the differen-tial score approach in test interpretation, since the relative attainment of "normal" levels of performance within categories of abilities such as those suggested in Table 1 can be quite useful with regard to the determination of rather more subtle and im-portant dimensions of brain-behavior relationships than those that can be considered within the brain damage vs. no brain damage dichotomy.

Pathognomonic signs. This essentially qualitative approach to the interpretation of neuropsychological test data can also be quantified, at least to a certain extent. A sign, by its very nature, is either present or absent (at least if we disregard the mythical "soft" signs of those who are committed to the syndrome of minimal brain dysfunction). In this sense, it is not amenable to analysis as a continuous variable. However, it is possible to determine the absolute or proportional frequency of occurrence of a particular sign in an individual's behavioral repertoire. This is the approach that Sweeney and Rourke (1978) used in the classification of disabled spellers into those who were "phonetically accurate" and those who were "phonetically inaccurate."

In the latter study, comparisons were made between disabled spellers who were equated with respect to their impaired level of performance in spelling, but who differed markedly in the levels of phonetic accuracy exhibited in the words that they misspelled. The key to the success of this study was the development of a system that enabled the investigators to specify, in an absolutely reliable fashion, the phonetic accuracy of each of the disabled speller's misspelled words on a syllable-by-syllable basis. Subsequent studies in this series have attested to the reliability and validity of the separation of groups on this basis (Rourke, 1983; Sweeney & Rourke, in press).

In the present context, the principal point of interest with respect to the data of these investigations is that this index of phonetic inaccuracy (shown in these studies to be associated with a wide variety of psycholinguistic and other higher-order adaptive deficiencies) can be quantified in a reliable fashion. Indeed, the controversy surrounding the use of such an index and the sometimes conflicting results obtained by investigators who were employing it would appear to be related to the fact that they depended upon the rating of each misspelled word as a whole and on a qualitative basis, thus rendering the reliability of measurement of the principal variable of interest (i.e., phonetic accuracy) considerably less than perfect. The system employed by Sweeney and Rourke was not subject to such problems, since each misspelled syllable was simply compared to all possible graphic equivalents of it for the determination of whether or not the syllable was spelled in a phonetically accurate manner. The minimization of error with respect to the independent (or control) variable in this series of investigations was probably responsible for their very clear-cut and largely unambiguous results.

The clarity with which this "sign" could be quantified would also suggest that other such "signs," be they of the aphasiological variety or not, would be amenable to more satisfactory types of neuropsychological analysis were they to be couched in such terms. Certainly, attempts to frame decision rules on an actuarial basis would be aided inestimably thereby.

Differential score approach. As suggested above, the actuarial approach to the analysis of quantitative data is particularly suited to the application of the differential score interpretation strategy. In this approach to interpretation, the clinician pays particular attention to differences in levels of performances on selected tests and measures rather than to their absolute levels. At the same time, there are a number of ways in which differences between performances of children can be characterized. At its simplest level, the differential score approach involves the specification of the difference between two particular scores. Another way of approaching the same question that may yield different results, however, is to compare these two scores with respect to their deviations from the developmental norms for the tests in question. The situation becomes more complex when one wishes to consider simultaneously the relative differences between any particular score and a large number of scores with respect to their deviations from one another and their deviations from developmental norms. Even more complexity obtains if one wishes to express these sets of differences in terms of standard score units and centiles and other metrics for particular purposes, or if one wishes to transform particular sets of scores into composite indices (e.g., motor skills, sensory-perceptual skills) for the purpose of sequential comparisons of these composite scores.

It should be obvious that none but the most simple levels of these comparisons can be carried out with ease by the clinician unless he/she has access to an actuarial program for their determination. Furthermore, it should be clear that the extent to which each of these scores, composite or otherwise, can be quantified constitutes the extent to which actuarial algorithms can be used to aid in the process.

Comparisons of performance on the two sides of the body. Another type of differential score comparison is that which involves systematic comparisons of motor, psychomotor, and sensory-perceptual performances on the two sides of the body. Here, the relative merits of the automated approach to systematic comparisons are exactly the same as they are for the differential scores approach. An example of how multiple comparisons within the motor and sensory-perceptual realms can be fruitful with respect to the correlates of neurological disease in adults is a recent study by Hom and Reitan (1982). Similar comparisons have been made with children (Rourke & Strang, 1978; Rourke & Telegdy, 1971), and their relevance to assessment considerations has been outlined elsewhere (Rourke, 1981, 1982b; Rourke et al., 1983).

Subtype classification. Finally, a relatively new variety of assessment strategy is emerging in conjunction with the application of numerical taxonomy techniques to the classification of children with neuropsychological disorders. So far, the determination of subtypes has been largely confined to attempts at the classification of children with various types of learning disabilities (e.g., Doehring, Trites, Parel, & Fiedoriwicz, 1981; Morris, Blashfield, & Satz, 1981; Petrauskas & Rourke, 1979; Rourke, in press). However, there is every reason to believe that this type of classification exercise will be applied to children with a variety of disorders of neuropsychological significance.

At least potentially, these techniques of classification have considerable relevance for the assessment, habilitation, and rehabilitation of children who are suffering from cerebral dysfunction. With respect to the application of these techniques to children with learning disabilities, it is clear that classification can be carried out in a reliable fashion. What remains to be done is to demonstrate that these reliable classifications have some external validity. (Once again, we see that the progression of psychological inquiry in this field began with the question of reliability and then moved on to the consideration of issues of concurrent and predictive validity.) The next task in the process is to determine whether children so classified are more or less amenable to distinct intervention strategies. In the case of learning disabilities, there is emerging evidence that at least some of the reliable subtypes identified are valid from a concurrent standpoint (e.g., Fletcher, in press; Lovrich & Stamm, 1983), and that various intervention strategies are differentially effective with them (e.g, Lyon, in press). The latter type of evidence, of course, speaks to the issue of the predictive validity of these subtypes.

The relevance of these findings to the topic under immediate discussion is quite straightforward. The statistical and mathematical techniques involved in numeric taxonomy are exceedingly complex. Their use for clinical purposes would be greatly enhanced by the application of actuarial decision-making models in the individual case for the determination of subtype membership. This can only be done if the data are quantifiable and if exactly the same tests and measures have been administered in the standardized manner to the children in question. Even fairly minor deviations from standardized testing conditions, and any deviations whatsoever with respect to the tests and measures employed, would vitiate this entire effort. This does not mean that only one battery of tests or only one set of testing conditions should be employed by child neuropsychologists. All it does mean is that the taxonomic techniques will not work for any situation other than one exactly identical to that upon which the taxonomy was derived. Let us be quick to add, however, that this is simply a reflection of the current state of affairs. It is at least potentially possible that the creative use of well-designed factorial dimensions and other data reduction techniques will allow for the rather more general applicability of such subtyping procedures to assessment modes that are quite different from those upon which the taxonomy was originally derived.

STATISTICAL APPROACHES TO QUANTITATIVE ASSESSMENT

Given the above considerations, we turn now to the examination of a number of appropriate statistical methods for research designed to improve the validity of neuropsychological assessment data. A number of representative techniques will be considered that are applicable for the treatment of data derived from neuropsychological assessments of children.

In presenting certain statistical techniques, we do not imply that these are methods to be preferred in any data reduction within the scope of children's studies. Rather, these techniques are presented because they combine various strengths in description, prediction and theory development. In addition, our selection has been made with special attention to the potential of the techniques to identify and explicate subtypes in children with learning disabilities and/or frank neurological deficits.

We should also note that our consideration here is restricted to multivariate techniques. This is appropriate, given the multidimensionality of the skills of interest and their relationship to brain functioning. As such, the traditional bivariate laboratory experiment appears to have approached its useful limit as a principal basis for the understanding of children's central processing deficiencies. The complex and interdependent nature of disorders of reading, spelling, arithmetic, concept formation and other higher-order skills cannot be done justice in analysis without techniques that allow for the simultaneous evaluation of a number of behavioral parameters.

Our view is that the construction of cogent theory and reliable predictive technology in this area requires a careful sampling of abilities, as noted above. In a similar way, we see the application of various analysis techniques as specific in aim and sequential in their deployment. A premature use of certain methods is as likely to produce false leads as would the (inadvertent) restriction of variable range be likely to result in inadequate coverage.

Perhaps our objective is best served by presenting an overview of how multivariate techniques may be seen to relate to each other.

In Figure 1 (adapted from Gordesch, Katschnig, & Poldinger, 1973) we see a direct comparison of the relative merits of various techniques of statistical analysis. Plus (+) symbols denote positive capabilities, while minus (−) symbols denote lack of capability to achieve the objective in question. Key features relevant to the evaluation, construction, and validation of typologies are considered. It can be seen most readily that no single technique provides for all objectives, and certain aspects of the underlying distribution of data or the statistical model may be inconsistent with the researcher's goals.

It may be useful to review each of these techniques with special reference to their role in a research strategy for children with learning disabilities.

	Evaluation of a priori typology	Construction of new typology of persons	Assignment of new person to given typology	Model for two variables	Type of data	Normal distribution necessary
Discriminant analysis	+ + +	−	+ + +	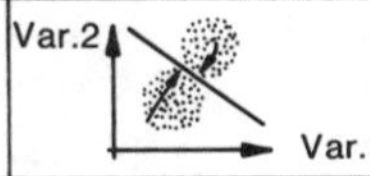 Var.2 ... Var.1	Quantitative (qualitative)	+/(−)
Profile analysis	+ + +	−	−	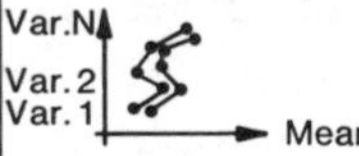 Var.N Var.2 Var.1 ... Mean	Quantitative or qualitative	−
Factor analysis	−	+[1]	+	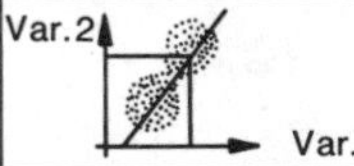 Var.2 ... Var.1	Quantitative (qualitative)	+/(−)
Cluster analysis	−	+ +	+ +/−[2]	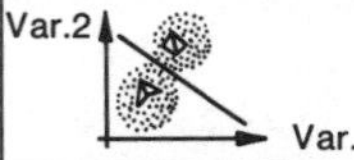 Var.2 ... Var.1	Quantitative or qualitative	−
Conditional cluster analysis	−	+ + +[3]	+ +	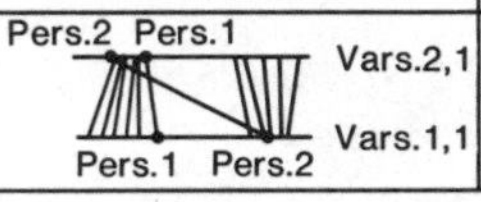 Pers.2 Pers.1 ... Vars.2,1 Vars.1,1 Pers.1 Pers.2	Quantitative or qualitative	+/−[2]

1 +++ FOR typology of variables ("dimensional structure")
2 Depends on method
3 Two sets of data necessary (e.g. somatic and psychic)

Fig. 1

Discriminant analysis is a most powerful method for the optimal determination of the distance separation between two or more groups across a number of variables (Adams, 1979; Fletcher, Rice, & Ray, 1978). A variety of techniques have been described for the manipulation of multivariate vectors of scores so as to produce the greatest mathematical (and perhaps psychological) distance as a result of the application of an empirically derived equation. Usually, the procedure is conducted on a linear combination of variables, but this need not be the case.

In studies of children's learning disabilities, a common application of the discriminant analysis is the post-hoc examination of test data. Having done this, the discriminant analysis is carried out, with the results interpreted in terms of the relative importance of test variables, the neuropsychological test indices thought to be most salient for brain functions, or the relative potency of the test indices in prediction. This kind of utilization of discriminant analysis not only does not accomplish the stated objective, but fails to take advantage of the very strengths of the method.

Briefly stated, the place of discriminant analysis is usually at a later point in a research program. Once a typology or system for assessment and classification is created, the technique becomes a powerful tool to examine its potential and to test more crucially its predictive power through cross validation. Rarely should discriminant analysis be utilized in search of new typology, since chance combinations of unreliable distance differences between vectors and groups are weighted equally with real ones. A more detailed discussion of a plan for the use of this technique is available (Adams, 1979), which is readily supplemented by more detailed discussion in most comprehensive textbooks on multivariate analysis.

Profile analysis is a series of techniques designed, first, to create exemplars, and then to match individual protocols against them. That is, one must first develop a family of target profiles; following this, some method must be developed to evaluate the "fit" between the target profile and individual cases which are to be classified.

Every profile, or set of test variables, can be seen to have three types of information: elevation, scatter, and shape. We will review these briefly. Elevation corresponds to the overall level of performance and is easily conceived as the height of the particular test profile along the ordinate (y axis). In neuropsychological terms, this corresponds to the absolute level of various scores as seen in IQ or other variables (e.g., 70 Verbal IQ versus 100 versus 120, etc.). Scatter information is a term defining the variability of scores along the profile. The term is

often thought to have meaning in terms of psychological inconsistency, or perhaps in terms of stable limits or barriers to performance in certain psychological skills. Shape information is
that conception of the overall residual pattern or configuration,
once elevation and scatter have been removed.

Profile analysis is especially useful in advanced stages of
typology development, when very precise measures of similarity and
dissimilarity are of interest and the principal concerns of the
existence and reliability of the overall classification scheme
have been put to rest. Again, a serious error can occur if the
researcher should use the technique when its role is inappropriate. Some researchers eager to produce visual "subtypes" in their
data can create them because of the insensitivity of the technique
to misapplication. Later, the investigator will find his or her
new-found typologies to be unstable or only reflective of some
obvious parameters in the test ensemble (e.g., Verbal IQ versus
Performance IQ salience). The application of profile analysis in
the proper context is a rather direct exercise (see Neufeld, 1977,
p. 152-163) that has pleasing results when introduced at the appropriate point in the research program.

The previous discussion of discriminant analysis and profile
analysis illustrates the strong role these techniques play in the
examination of existing typologies. They are presented here first
because they are the most powerful statistically, most attuned to
the production of "confirmatory" evidence, and most vulnerable to
inopportune deployment. To emphasize again, the proper role for
these techniques is at a more mature time in the life of the
typological model. The following techniques enjoy the advantages
of being exploratory or descriptive techniques in the main, but
also have the capability to be employed as confirmatory strategies.

Factor analysis is perhaps the oldest, most intricate and
most versatile of the techniques in the multivariate armamentarium. To understand factor analysis we might first contrast its
objective with that of the standard techniques for variance analysis.

Statistical methods for analyzing sources of variation
amongst scores or indices exist in the univariate and multivariate
cases -- Analysis of Variance (ANOVA) and Multivariate Analysis of
Variance (MANOVA), respectively. These techniques are useful when
a distinction between independent and dependent variables exists.
In reality, analysis of variance techniques examine means of
scores -- or variability in mean scores relative to other sources
of variance. In the case of factor analysis, the independent-
dependent variable distinction fades. We operate in factor analysis by analyzing inter-relationships and mutual covariation around

the variables' theoretical averages (which are of no direct
interest in this technique).

It may be well to ask why one would seek to study systematically the variance sources in a matrix when all variables are
dependent? Put simply, factor analysis is a search for subsets of
variables or groupings that can serve to summarize existing interrelationships in the matrix and that often shed light on the unifying influences within and between these subsets. Obviously,
this can be a powerful technique when the investigator's departure
point is a rich array of test information or other indicators of
the child's performance. The prospect that the data can be understood in a multidimensional shorthand has appeal.

Factor analysis can shed light on the nature of the test
matrix, but is subject to limitations. Once understood, these
considerations can be put in their proper light and the full advantage of matrix reduction realized. One source of potential
problems is the nature of the metric used to depict the inter-
relationship of variables. The correlation coefficient is the
usual input to factor analysis. As such, the correlation coefficient represents a particular choice emphasizing scatter information and relegating elevation to a minor role. Generally, distance metrics do the reverse with data input to a factor analysis. Mixed or specially developed metrics may represent the way
to proceed in such cases where level of performance and subject
variability are thought to require equal play.

Another influence in the matrix is subject sampling. Because
the decision concerning inclusion of certain clinical groups and
controls affects the input matrix structure, it cannot help but
affect the factor analysis outcome. Often, the decision to
include certain subjects is taken because of a later expectation
that "factor scores" or linear representations of the factors will
create interesting differences between the original groups. This
is an example of a valid reason to include clinical cases and controls in such an analysis.

Additionally, the distributions of the original variables
will create certain impacts on the relationship metric between
variables and the input matrix. In particular, skewed and multi-
modal variables often seen in cognitive-perceptual-motor tasks
will produce artifactual results and even false factor extraction
in some cases.

Actual methods of factor analysis used in children's neuropsychological investigations vary and fall broadly into *principal
components* and *principal factors*. The components are true summary
transformations of the input matrix, or actually new dependent

variables fashioned directly from the input variables themselves. The components are direct and accurate successive summaries of the variance in the matrix, and can be used as intermediate variables when the goal is to use the principal components as a more manageable number of variables as input to another kind of procedure. An example of this is the work of Joschko and Rourke (in press) who used components as input to a cluster analysis as a classification strategy.

Principal factors can be thought of as factor analysis proper. In this technique, the analysis treats part of the variance in any variable as common (or shared) with other variables and part as unique. Many different procedures exist for the actual extraction of factors, procedures to "rotate" a solution to a final criterion, and their evaluation. In this connection, the important thing to remember is that a factor solution is only one of many possible solutions and that indeterminacy is an inherent feature of factor analysis.

Certain conventions exist in factor analysis, principally because the results that emerge when these conventions are in effect appear to make the most psychological sense. For example, in the study of intelligence test scores, most often it has been the case that a varimax rotation has been used with orthogonal factors. There is no compelling mathematical reason for this, except that the resultant psychological meaning of the factors seems satisfying and has been verified by others. In more recent times, opinion has shifted in favor of non-orthogonal factors as the best descriptors of the structure of psychological measures (Rummel, 1970).

Actually, most researchers see factor analysis as perforce being conducted on relationships between variables (R-type) or people (Q-type). In fact, these are only two of six potential combinations of relationships between tests, people, and observation intervals. It would appear that the full potential of factor analysis -- particularly in regard to the longitudinal dimension -- has not been tapped. For example, no factor analysis of the relationship between test-retest scores and people (summed over tests) or test-retest scores and tests (summed over people) has ever been reported in the areas of study under consideration here. Such an undertaking would require little missing data and a sampling of the test universe that would be robust.

It would be fair to suggest that factor analysis has many features and will use increasing use as an intermediate technique where the researcher/clinician wants to make the transition between the context of initial typology development and eventual validation.

Cluster analysis is the approach most frequently used in the multivariate reduction of neuropsychological data. In the area of subtype development, it certainly has merited study as an exploratory method. Morris et al. (1981) have described well the various approaches to clustering and the problems inherent in each.

For some, cluster analysis represents the best exploratory technique possible, because of the experimenter's ability to partition the variable space in creative ways in search of sensible subgroupings of subjects. It should be cautioned that this capability is only as good as the variable subset available for partition. That is, coverage becomes a crucial issue if the intent is to be able to (1) refer the typology back to the cerebral and developmental substrate, (2) analyze the psychometric and factorial structure of the correlation or distance matrix, and (3) use the variable array predictively and in a way acceptable as a standard for clinical practice.

At present, there is little evidence to suggest that cluster analysis and its near relative, Q-factor analysis, produce different initial typologies. For example, Del Dotto and Rourke (in press) have reported that their analysis of the same data using representative cluster analysis and Q-factor analysis produced 100 percent replication of subtypes.

Be that as it may, it is clear that the available methods for cluster analysis are as varied as are any in multivariate mathematics today. Based on an original compilation by the statistical research laboratory at the University of California, Berkeley, we present a current synopsis of computer software available for "cluster type" techniques. We should note that factor analysis is listed because of the belief by many analysts that it is, indeed, a variant of cluster analysis. For a fuller description of the intent of these clustering techniques, refer to Morris et al. (1981):

LISTING OF PROGRAMS BY ANALYSIS CATEGORY

1.   Cluster Analysis

     A.   ADDTREE
     B.   AGCLUS
     C.   ANDERBERG
     D.   BC-TRY
     E.   C-LAB
     F.   CLUSTAN
     G.   NI-PAK
     H.   SIMGRA
     I.   TAXON

2.   Factor Analysis, Ordination, and Related Techniques

   A.   BC-TRY
   B.   BMDP
   C.   COMPREY
   D.   SPSS
   E.   TAXON

3.   Multidimensional Scaling and Related Techniques

   A.   C-LAB (nonlinear mapping)
   B.   INDSCAL
   C.   MDSCAL-5M
   D.   PREFMAP
   E.   PROFIT
   F.   TORSCA8

4.   Character Correlation

   A.   CHA

5.   Geographic Variation Analysis

   A.   UNIVAR

6.   Cladistic Analysis

   A.   CLINCH
   B.   WAGNER

7.   Miscellaneous Programs

   A.   CLUMP
   B.   GENDIST

PROGRAM OUTLINES

1.   ADDTREE

ADDTREE is a program written by Sattath and Tversky to construct additive similarity trees (dendrograms) from proximity
data, and is viewed by them as having advantages over MDS and
agglomerative hierarchical clustering techniques (most of
which satisfy the highly restrictive "ultrametric inequal-
ity"). In ADDTREE dendrograms, the similarity of objects (or
variables) directly corresponds to the tree distance between
them. The program can handle over 200 objects or variables,
more on larger machines. Also see AGCLUS, which produces
similar dendrograms.

2.   AGCLUS

AGCLUS performs 7 varieties of agglomerative hierarchical cluster analysis (single and complete linkage, 4 types of average and centroid linkage, and Ward's minimum variance method) on similarity or dissimilarity matrices input to the program. The hierarchical structuring is shown in very clear line-printer-generated dendrograms (trees). See Sneath and Sokal (1973) for a discussion of these types of cluster analysis.

3.   ANDERBERG

ANDERBERG is a set of Fortran IV programs included by Anderberg in his book, **Cluster Analysis for Applications.** Programs included perform the following analyses: (1) partitioning interval variables into equal length categories; (2) computing matrices of association among interval variables, nominal variables, and mixtures thereof; (3) computing a wide variety of association measures among binary variables; (4) seven types of hierarchical cluster analysis (each via 3 different computational approaches); (5) four types of nearest centroid sorting (k-means methods) for nonhierarchical clustering; (6) various programs to aid in the interpretation of cluster analysis results.

4.   BC-TRY

BC-TRY is a large, versatile, integrated system for performing many types of MDA. Some of its procedures are as follows: (1) principal components analysis and many varieties of factor analysis; (2) collinearity cluster analysis of both variables and objects; (3) iterative partitioning clustering of objects (up to 5,000); (4) 3-space plots of both variables and objects; (5) comparative cluster analysis and matrix fitting procedures; (6) Tryon's nonlinear "typological" prediction of criterion variables.

5.   CHA

CHA performs an information theoretic analysis of character correlation for qualitative characters. Input is a rectangular matrix of objects by characters. Each pair or any combination of pairs of characters are analyzed. For each pair of characters compared, output includes: (1) a measure of similarity and dissimilarity; (2) unconditional and conditional probabilities of the states of each character; (3) unconditional and conditional entropies of each character; (4) entropy common to both characters; and, (5) the fraction of entropy of one character contained in the other.

6. **C-LAB**

C-LAB is an integrated, interactive program for performing a series of functions related to cluster analysis. C-LAB's excellent graphics may be routed to a graphics display terminal, and its plotter-drawn graphs and diagrams are of publication-level quality. Some of its features are as follows: (1) seven standard measures of similarity and distance, plus Minkowski distances in general; (2) principal components analysis and nonlinear mapping, with 2- and 3-space plots; (3) five methods of agglomerative hierarchical clustering, plus the drawing of minimum spanning trees; (4) k-means clustering; (5) representation of data in up to 18 dimensions by computer-drawn (Chernoff) faces. Sneath and Sokal (1973) provide a good introductory discussion of most of these techniques.

7. **CLINCH**

CLINCH is a program for constructing estimates of evolutionary history by the determination of sets or cliques of mutually compatible characters. In its basic mode of operation, it accepts as input a set of hypothesized character state trees and a data matrix and produces as output a compatibility matrix, a list of cliques, and phylogenetic trees based upon the largest cliques. Optionally, it can function as a stand-alone clique finder or as a stand-alone tree constructor.

8. **CLUMP**

CLUMP is a small program which discovers monothetic subsets of objects within an object-by-character matrix. The subsets are listed by object name in alphabetic order, by character in alphabetic order or numeric order, by size and number of shared characters.

9. **CLUSTAN**

CLUSTAN, like BC-TRY, is a large, integrated system, but is primarily oriented toward the cluster analysis of objects and variables. In comparison to other MDA programs, CLUSTAN has the advantage of being able to handle large numbers of variables (200 continuous, 400 binary) and has a large number of options for measuring similarity between objects or variables, similarity between clusters, and the overall homogeneity of a classification. Some of its other procedures are the following: (1) eight methods of agglomerative hierarchical clustering; (2) a generalized partitioning method, optimizing any one of 14 between-cluster similarity measures;

(3) monothetic divisive clustering; and, (4) minimum spanning
tree partitioning. Wishart (1978) includes both a theoretical discussion of these methods and procedures for using the
programs.

10. COMREY

COMREY is a set of programs written by Comrey. Programs
included perform the following functions or analyses: (1) raw
item scoring to form composites, and conversion of these to
centile or standardized T scores; (2) scatter plots of
selected variables, to show possible nonlinear relationships;
(3) factor extraction by principal axes or minimum residual
methods, with Varimax rotation; (4) orthogonal analytic rotations using Comrey's "tandem criteria" methods and analytic
oblique rotations; (5) **hand** rotations, with 2-space plots of
selected factors.

11. GENDIST

GENDIST is a small program for calculating genetic distance
between populations using the formulations of Nei and of
Rogers for allozyme data. Input is a matrix of allozyme fre-
quencies for a series of populations. Output can be punched
or printed distance matrices and associated statistics.

12. MDS-UW

MDS-UW is a set of programs for performing a variety of multidimensional scaling (MDS) and related techniques. Programs
included are the following: (1) TORSCA 8 (Torgerson metric &
nonmetric MDS); (2) MDSCAL 5M (Kruskal's nonmetric MDS); (3)
INDSCAL (scaling of proximities data, retaining individual
differences); (4) PREFMAP (or, UNFOLD) (metric & nonmetric
generalizations of Coomb's unfolding model); (5) PROFIT
(fitting of property vectors into stimulus spaces); (6) C-
MATCH (orthogonal matrix fitting); (7) MONOTONE (monotone
analysis of variance); (8) NMREG (nonmetric regression).
These programs have been used intramurally at the University
of Washington but may be available for external use soon.

13. NT-PAK

NT-PAK is composed of a series of programs for cluster analysis. The package contains a number of programs of various
levels of sophistication. The tasks performed by this series
of programs are as follows: (1) testing of characters for
skewness and kurtosis; (2) computation of several similarity
and distance measures; (3) hierarchical cluster analysis,
including the map cluster analysis of Carmichael; (4) cal-

culation of cophenetic correlation coefficients; and (5) matrix inversion. Sneath and Sokal (1973) discuss these types of methods. This package parallels what is contained in CLUSTAN, but NT-PAK is less inclusive.

14. ORDIFLEX

ORDIFLEX is a flexible program for four ordination procedures: weighted averages, polar (Bray-Curtis) ordination, principal components analysis, and reciprocal averaging. Used primarily for ecological studies, the input is typically a species-by-samples matrix. Options for graphic output of ordination are available. The user manual to be released will outline both the theory and recommendations for use of the program.

15. SIMGRA

SIMGRA calculates the generalized simple matching coefficient of Estabrook and Rogers and performs a graph theoretic single-link hierarchical cluster analysis on the resultant similarity matrix. Input is an object-by-character matrix. Output includes the following: (1) the similarity matrix; (2) a table of order similarities; (3) the results of graph partitioning; and, (4) nodal distance arrays.

16. TAXON(LANCE)

TAXON is a set of pattern analysis programs developed under the direction of G.N. Lance at CSIRO in Canberra City, Australia. The programs cover three types of classification strategies: polythetic divisive. Some programs accept only binary data, some only numeric, but at least two (MULTBET and REMUL) will accept any combination of the following types of attributes: disordered multistate, ordered multistate and continuous (numerical). TAXON includes three ordination programs, performing principal components analysis, principal co-ordinates analysis, and canonical analysis, among other techniques. See Sneath and Sokal (1973) for a discussion of some of Lance's techniques.

17. UNIVAR

UNIVAR performs Gabriel's sum of squares test procedure on ranked means in order to examine patterns of geographic variation. Options include the calculation of means, standard deviations and other statistics for each sample and each character, and regressions of means.

18. **WAGNER**

>   WAGNER calculates evolutionary trees which are the most par-
>   simonious for the data at hand. A tree will be calculated
>   from either raw data or from a distance matrix. Other
>   options are as follows: (1) analysis of length of user-
>   inputted trees; (2) rooting of tree at midpoint between two
>   most distant taxa; (3) generation of a homoplasy matrix; (4)
>   output of character data for hypothetical ancestors; (5)
>   ranges, patristic lengths, and consistency indices of the
>   characters; (6) a list of shared character states for each
>   taxon; and, (7) a list of changes in each character.

This array of programs should give some indication of the potential for exploratory work in multivariate analysis of data from
quantitative neuropsychological approaches. If the data input is
equal to this cornucopia of statistical programs, the possible
gains in understanding of central processing deficits in children
are considerable.

A REVIEW AND EXAMPLES OF PROBLEM FANTASIES

A careful reviewing of Figure 1 at this point should resensi-
tize the reader to the interdependency of these techniques and the
need to consider carefully the timing of their deployment in the
reduction of data. Perhaps the most common failures of multivariate methods occur because of misconceptions concerning the role
and yield of the methods. As an example, we present the three
"fantasies" that seem to be the driving force behind the majority
of misapplications of multivariate techniques:

FANTASY 1 - MULTIVARIATE STATISTICS WILL TELL ME THE UNDERLYING STRUCTURE OF MY DATA AND SHOW ME WHAT IS IMPORTANT

In factor analysis, this takes the form of a notion that the
"real" abilities underlying some group of measures will be
apparent. A variant of this conclusion is the certainty that the
number of factors extracted has something to do with the number of
psychological functions being examined by the set of measures. In
truth, this is a miscalculation. Factor analysis turns out to be
no better than the variables put into it. Their nature and distribution must be carefully considered. If one includes many measures of the same thing (e.g., motor behavior) or uses highly
intercorrelated data for some function, it should be no surprise
when a factor pops out which "looks like" that function. As mentioned above, if the variables which go in have unusual distributions, strange things will also happen. What factor analysis can
do is to make clear the essential dimensionality of the data.
This means that the interrelationships between the variables can
be summarized in a parsimonious way, thus affording the opportun-

ity to view the problems from a new vantage point. Interpretation of one's factor analysis and the use of factor scores in neuropsychological research should be done carefully, and not in the hope of finding an easy route through complex data. Factor scores are really second-order extrapolations from the original data, with an entire set of problems and properties of their own.

FANTASY 2 - MULTIVARIATE TECHNIQUES WILL ENABLE ME TO SELECT A BEST SET OF PREDICTORS FROM AMONGST MANY

In test battery research, this means we can retain the first few tests and dispose of the rest. This is usually a discriminant function or regression fantasy, and involves some need to show clinical accuracy. Such problems as methodological variance, suppressor or moderator variables, and replicability are not usually given the attention that they merit. The interesting thing is that techniques such as discriminant function have little to do with clinical neuropsychological utility anyway -- only one aspect of the data (level of performance) is employed in what is really a complex maximization problem. This technique assumes that the dependent criterion group variable is reliably and validly defined, which is yet another act of faith in most instances. Even if one accepts this definition of dependent criterion group membership, the discriminant function only tells one the maximum degree of separation between groups, and the likely results in the individual case. In neuropsychological research, the principal interest is often focused on the off-diagonal elements where prediction and "reality" do not agree. Thus, in the strict sense, discriminant analysis is only one method in the development of clinical classification schema.

In stepwise approaches in regression and discriminant analysis, the notion of variable entry order as indicative of the relative predictive importance of a measure has been stated in print and repeated so many times that it is assumed by many to be fact. Statistical experts do not consider this to be as true as computer manual writers would believe in their instructions to potential users. Actually, the non-stepwise method has a great deal to offer and has a much more solid base of statistical knowledge behind it.

FANTASY 3 - THE USE OF MULTIVARIATE STATISTICS RELIEVES ONE OF THE NEED TO STUDY THE INDIVIDUAL VARIABLE DISTRIBUTIONS AND RELATIONSHIPS BECAUSE VECTORS OF SCORES ARE TREATED SIMULTANEOUSLY

This is a particularly tough one, since it is, in one sense, true. In general, though, the use of these techniques requires even *more* intimate knowledge of interrelationships and distributions. In neuropsychological areas, our emphasis on temporal measurement as well as the impaired populations we often study almost guarantees problems of skewness as well as other anomalies which will affect the multivariate outcome. Individual variable scatterplots and crosstabulations should be studied assiduously for those anomalies such as heteroskedasticity and other phenomena. We all learned that these make a difference in univariate research; we should also be aware that they make a difference in the multivariate case.

Many of these fantasies are born of experience in using computer manuals, programs and facilities. As a positive step, we present some guidelines for clinical researchers who are contemplating a multivariate analysis of their data to be conducted on the modal university computing environment.

1. Read and learn the overall mechanics of the multivariate techniques you will use. Go beyond the programming manuals and obtain the statistical references they cite, and add your own. Ask your statistical colleagues for information and remind them that your background is not in advanced mathematics. They almost always will help. Do not be put off by seeming complexity.

    In doing this, you will be surprised by the glibness with which serious and controversial problems are treated in programming manuals. Granted, one may have to learn a bit along the way. It is not that bad, though, and you will gain new power over your own data. Most investigators are dedicated to the notion that the brain is not a "black box," so why should a man-made machine and its algorithms deter us?

    In dealing with consultants and other computer minions, one should insist on full explanations and competent solutions -- and then expect to pay for it. Like your clinical or professional opinion, it is a service, and we all know what nearly free advice on brain functions is worth.

2. Trust nothing you read from your printed computer outputs without cross-checking on another algorithm and reconciling both programs. You may be surprised to see the differences between major program packages which purport to do the same thing.

3. Collect documentation and error notices carefully. Most major computer centers and package producers have update services. Often, the notices are statements of flaws or mistakes in the manual or program. The computer age has brought us a new anxiety for the graduate student and investigator -- the real prospect that a computer error will invalidate the dissertation or research project. This need not happen with a

healthy dose of intellectual curiosity and cautious cross-calculation.

4.   Set a course and keep it. Decide on what analyses you expect
     to do and why; then, stick to your plan. If your results are
     less than spectacular in terms of prediction or solution,
     carefully study what happened. Above all, resist the temp-
     tation to treat the computer like a video game, putting in
     coins until your score gets high enough. A reanalysis should
     be done with good reasons in mind and a thorough understand-
     ing of what has already happened.

5.   If possible, check your solutions against previously pub-
     lished multivariate work using the same kind of data. If
     your results are comparable (at least roughly), it is another
     piece of possible convergent validity.

In this chapter, we have attempted to present the methodological
framework for advancing the quantitative assessment of neuropsychological functions in the child. We started from an articulated
rationale for variable selection, deployment of assessment
resources, and a conceptual model for the understanding of the
interdependency of brain functions. Successful application of
these principles will produce a rich test array equal to the
understanding of questions of importance in child neuropsychology
today. The relationship of this test array to the powerful multivariate methods currently available was presented, along with an
appreciation of the need for application of the methods, in a dis-
ciplined and logical fashion. Given proper deployment of these
techniques at the proper time, the full power of the original data
may be realized. This would complete an internally consistent
process of planning, data collection and data analysis and would
be expected to lead to new planning based upon a quantitative and
public process of inquiry -- open for any to pursue.

REFERENCES

Adams, K.M. Linear discriminant analysis in clinical neuropsy-
     chology research. **Journal of Clinical Neuropsychology**, 1979,
     1, 259-272.
Anderberg, M.R. **Cluster analysis for applications.** New York:
     Academic Press, 1973.
Benton, A.L. **Sentence memory test.** Iowa City, Iowa, Author,
     1965.
Del Dotto, J.E., & Rourke, B.P. Subtypes of left-handed learning
     disabled children. In B.P. Rourke (Ed.), **Learning disabili-
     ties in children: Advances in subtype analysis.** New York:
     Guilford, in press.
Doehring, D.C. **Patterns of impairment in specific reading dis-
     ability.** Bloomington: Indiana University Press, 1968.

Doehring, D.G., Trites, R.L., Patel, P.G., & Fiedorowicz, A.M. **Reading disabilities: The interaction of reading, language, and neuropsychological deficits.** New York: Academic Press, 1981.

Dunn, L.M. **Expanded manual for the Peabody Picture Vocabulary Test.** Circle Pines, Minnesota: American Guidance Service, 1965.

Fletcher, J.M. Behavioral and electrophysiological validation studies of learning disability subtypes. In B.P. Rourke (Ed.), **Learning disabilities in children: Advances in subtype analysis.** New York: Guilford, in press.

Fletcher, J., Rice, W., & Ray, R. Linear discriminant function analysis in neuropsychology: Some uses and abuses. **Cortex,** 1978, **14,** 564–577.

Fletcher, J.M., & Satz, P. Developmental changes in the neuropsychological correlates of reading achievement: A six-year longitudinal follow-up. **Journal of Clinical Neuropsychology,** 1980, **2,** 23–37.

Goldberg, E., & Costa, L.D. Hemisphere differences in the acquisition and use of descriptive systems. **Brain and Language,** 1981, **14,** 144–173.

Gordesch, J., Katschnig, H., Poldinger, W., & Sint, P. Correlations between psychic and somatic symptoms in depression. In P. Kielholz (Ed.), **Masked depression.** Bern: Hans Huber, 1973.

Hom, J., & Reitan, R.M. Effects of lateralized cerebral damage upon contralateral and ipsilateral sensorimotor performances. **Journal of Clinical Neuropsychology,** 1982, **4,** 249–268.

Joschko, M., & Rourke, B.P. Subtypes of learning disabled children who exhibit the WISC ACID pattern. In B.P. Rourke (Ed.), **Learning disabilities in children: Advances in subtype analysis.** New York: Guilford, in press.

Kass, C.E. Auditory Closure Test. In J.J. Olsen & J.L. Olsen (Eds.), **Validity studies on the Illinois Test of Psycholinguistic Abilities.** Madison, Wisconsin: Photo Press, 1964.

Lovrich, D., & Stamm, J.S. Event-related potential and behavioral correlates of attention and reading retardation. **Journal of Clinical Neuropsychology,** 1983, **5,** 13–37.

Luria, A.R., & Majovski, L.V. Basic approaches used in American and Soviet clinical neuropsychology. **American Psychologist,** 1977, **32,** 959–968.

Lyon, R. Educational validation studies of learning disability subtypes. In B.P. Rourke (Ed.), **Learning disabilities in children: Advances in subtype analysis.** New York: Guilford, in press.

Morris, R., Blashfield, R., & Satz, P. Neuropsychology and cluster analysis: Potentials and problems. **Journal of Clinical Neuropsychology,** 1981, **3,** 79–99.

Neufeld, R.W.J. **Clinical quantitative methods.** New York: Grune and Stratton, 1977.

Pajurkova, E., Orr, R.R.,Rourke, B.P., & Finlayson, A.J. Children's Word-Finding Test: A verbal problem-solving task. **Perceptual and Motor Skills,** 1976, 42, 851–858.

Petrauskas, R.J., & Rourke, B.P. Identification of subgroups of retarded readers: A neuropsychological, multivariate approach. **Journal of Clinical Neuropsychology,** 1979, 1, 17–37.

Reitan, R.M. A research program on the psychological effects of brain lesions in human beings. In N.R. Ellis (Ed.), **International review of research in mental retardation.** Vol. 1. New York: Academic Press, 1966.

Reitan, R.M. Psychological effects of cerebral lesions in children of early school age. In R.M. Reitan & L.A. Davison (Eds.), **Clinical neuropsychology: Current status and applications.** Washington, D. C.: V.H. Winston & Sons, 1974.

Rourke, B.P. Brain-behavior relationships in children with learning disabilities: A research program. **American Psychologist,** 1975, **30,** 911–920.

Rourke, B.P. Issues in the neuropsychological assessment of children with learning disabilities. **Canadian Psychological Review,** 1976, **19,** 89–102.

Rourke, B.P. Reading, spelling, arithmetic disabilities: A neuropsychologic perspective. In H.R. Myklebust (Ed.), **Progress in learning disabilities.** Vol. IV. New York: Grune & Stratton, 1978.

Rourke, B.P. Neuropsychological assessment of children with learning disabilities. In S.B. Filskov & T.J. Boll (Eds.), **Handbook of clinical neuropsychology.** New York: Wiley-Interscience, 1981.

Rourke, B.P. Central processing deficiencies in children: Toward a developmental neuropsychological model. **Journal of Clinical Neuropsychology,** 1982, 4, 1–18. (a)

Rourke, B.P. Child-clinical neuropsychology: Assessment and intervention with the disabled child. In J. deWit & A.L. Benton (Eds.), **Perspectives in child study: Integration of theory and practice.** Lisse, The Netherlands: Swets & Zeitlinger, 1982. (b)

Rourke, B.P. Reading and spelling disabilities: A developmental neuropsychological perspective. In U. Kirk (Ed.), **Neuropsychology of language, reading, and spelling.** New York: Academic Press, 1983.

Rourke, B.P. (Ed.) **Learning disabilities in children: Advances in subtype analysis.** New York: Guilford, in press.

Rourke, B.P., Bakker, D.J., Fisk, J.L., & Strang, J.D. **Child neuropsychology.** New York: Guilford, 1983.

Rourke, B.P., & Orr, R.R. Prediction of the reading and spelling performances of normal and retarded readers: Four-year followup. **Journal of Abnormal Child Psychology**, 1978, 3, 62–66.

Rourke, B.P., & Telegdy, G.A. Lateralizing significance of WISC verbal-performance discrepancies for older children with learning disabilities. **Perceptual and Motor Skills**, 1971, **33**, 875–883.

Rummel, R.J. **Applied factor analysis.** Evanston: Northwestern University Press, 1970.

Sneath, P.H.A., & Sokal, R.R. **Numerical taxonomy: The principles and practice of numerical classification.** San Francisco: W.H. Freeman, 1973.

Sweeney, J.E., & Rourke, B.P. Neuropsychological significance of phonetically accurate and phonetically inaccurate spelling errors in younger and older retarded spellers. **Brain and Language**, 1978, **6**, 212–225.

Sweeney, J.E., & Rourke, B.P. Subtypes of spelling disabilities. In B.P. Rourke (Ed.), **Learning disabilities in children: Advances in subtype analysis.** New York: Guilford, in press.

Wishart, D. **Clustan User Manual.** Edinburgh: Edinburgh University Program Library Unit, 1978.

MENTAL RETARDATION

Gregory T. Slomka and Ralph E. Tarter

Department of Psychiatry
University of Pittsburgh School of Medicine
Pittsburgh, Pennsylvania

The diagnostic category, mental retardation, encompasses an extremely heterogeneous population. Well over two hundred causes of mental retardation have been identified. Genetics, inborn errors of metabolism, infection, trauma, anoxia, and prematurity are some of the more common etiological factors. Because mental retardation is a developmental disorder, the effects of the various etiological factors may not be detected until long after their initial impact on the developing organism. Indeed, more often than not there is no specific etiological event that is identifiable, nor can a particular event be inferred in most cases to have had a direct causal influence.

It is also important to note that mental retardation cannot be studied outside the context of the organism's ongoing process of development and differentiation in interacting with the environment. Therefore, it is not surprising that mental retardation can be manifest in a variety of forms. Further complicating the problem is the fact that mental retardation often occurs in association with other neurological and psychiatric disorders. These conditions include autism, psychosis, epilepsy, specific sensory deficits, and cerebral palsy; conditions which in themselves are associated with significant neuropsychological sequelae. Given these considerations, the description of the neuropsychological correlates of mental retardation constitute an exceedingly complex and challenging undertaking.

The following discussion will examine the specific contribution that clinical neuropsychology can make in improving the evaluation process, and in describing the cognitive and behavioral impairments associated with mental retardation. Neuropsychology, simply defined, is the study of brain-behavior relationships. from the observation of behavior under controlled test conditions, inferences can be made concerning the status of neurological functioning. To this extent, a comprehensive neuropsychological assessment constitutes a somewhat unique technology which surpasses the range of clinically relevant information that can be obtained from a routine psychometric assessment of intelligence and adaptive behavior.

Before addressing the specifics of the neuropsychological evaluation, it is first necessary, however, to consider certain conceptual and definitional issues germane to mental retardation. By first examining the evolutionary development of this diagnostic construct, the unique perspective that clinical neuropsychology can offer in the assessment and description of these syndromes will subsequently be better appreciated.

HISTORICAL DEVELOPMENT OF THE MENTAL RETARDATION CONSTRUCT

The definition and classification of mental retardation has, during the past several decades, undergone a number of changes reflecting, in general, the prevailing *Zeitgeist* of medical and psychological opinion. From an essentially biological or medical orientation, emphasizing etiological determinants, classification and definition has shifted to the current behavioral orientation which instead emphasizes the individual's functional capacities. The most current conceptual framework is epitomized in the latest edition of the American Psychiatric Association's Diagnostic and Statistical Manual (DSM III) (1980), in which mental retardation is diagnosed if the individual presents with significantly sub-average intellectual functioning accompanied by deficits in adaptive behavior, and an onset prior to eighteen years of age. This classification scheme, except for its reference to onset during the developmental period, all but excludes consideration of the biological development of the individual or etiological factors. In contrast, diagnosis utilizing either the preceding edition of the Diagnostic and Statistical Manual (DSM II) (1968), or that utilized in the *Manual on Terminology on Classification in Mental Retardation* (1977), a medical classification system, is based on etiological criteria; that is, mental retardation is categorized according to the causes of the syndrome. The various etiological categories are listed in Table 1.

A three digit code is applied to each category to signify the present level of mental retardation (mild - profound), regardless of whether the etiology is known or not. It is of interest to note that while the taxonomy is oriented toward etiological issues, the first seven categories implicate causal factors stemming from primary or secondary insult to the central nervous system. Despite variations and the multiplicity of the causal

Table 1. Mental retardation nomenclature medical classifications

.0   Following infections and intoxications

.1   Following trauma or physical agent

.2   With disorders of metabolism or nutrition

.3   Associated with gross brain disease (postnatal)

.4   Associated with diseases and conditions due to unknown prenatal influence

.5   With chromosomal abnormality

.6   Gestational disorders

.7   Following psychiatric disorder

.8   Environmental influences

.9   Associated with other conditions

pathways, however, the ultimate consequence is the same; namely, cerebral damage or dysfunction.

Although the pendulum has shifted to a behavioral classification, it would appear that each of the two systems are complementary in furthering our understanding of the mentally retarded. Note in Table 2 how the two approaches, representing different disciplines and each possessing specialized assessment tools, can be conjointly utilized from the perspective of a comprehensive evaluation. Since neuropsychology is the study of brain-behavior relationships, and is ideally suited to being amenable to clinical efforts from each of these two seemingly different perspectives, it offers a means to examine mental retardation from the standpoint of the medical model, in that it focuses on aspects of brain function, structure, and systemic interrelatedness; and in so doing, additionally derives detailed information about behavioral status. Thus, neuropsychology, by addressing the biological substrate, but also using behavioral measures, bridges the differences between these two divergent positions. This mutually inclusive perspective holds the promise of diminishing what has, up to now, been a wide schism between medically and behaviorally oriented practitioners.

For well over a century the etiology of mental retardation has been viewed dichotomously. Various classifications, such as "exogenous versus endogenous," "functional versus organic," and "brain damaged versus cultural familial" have been proposed. Pre-

Table 2. Models of descriptive process in mental retardation

Biological Bio-Medical Model	Behavioral Model
Causal Orientation	Descriptive Orientation
Neurology-Medicine	Psychology-Education
Laboratory & Medical Studies	Psychological & Functional
Diagnostic Statement	Assessment
	Behavioral Statement

dominant clinical lore has generally adopted the view that mentally retarded individuals can be divided into two groups – those
with a functional etiology, and those with an organic etiology.
This latter dichotomy is a source of active debate among researchers, and is essentially reduced to the question of whether all
mentally retarded persons manifest some form of brain pathology.
Adherents to the dichotomy position argue that even among individuals with an IQ below 50, only 10%-20% have brain pathology.
The remaining 80%-90% of retardates are believed to consist of
persons whose etiology derives from cultural, familial or other
unknown causes, or who have pathology that is not detectable by
current techniques. The opposing view holds that all individuals
who exhibit significantly subaverage intellectual performance
scores are neurologically impaired. If one operates from the
assumption that intact central nervous system functioning is a
requisite to higher order cognitive and intellectual functioning,
then to the extent that any of these processes are impaired, there
must be some corresponding deficit in the underlying neural substrate (Tredgold & Soddy, 1963; Masland, 1958).

A considerable literature exists indicating that there is a
much higher prevalence of brain pathology associated with mental
retardation than has been generally suspected. The post-mortem
neuropathological studies of Crome (1960), Malamud (1964), and
Jellinger (1972) conducted on institutionalized populations, have
consistently revealed the presence of cerebral pathology in over
90% of cases. These studies, despite their limitations in gen-
eralizing to the *in vivo* status of the patient, and the fact that
they were limited to institutionalized samples, nonetheless
illustrates that even for persons whose level of functioning was
in the mild to borderline range of mental retardation, that there
is evidence of neuropathology. However, it is noteworthy that
there were also exceptions. Some individuals who functioned in
the severe range of mental retardation showed little or no

discernible cerebral pathology. Thus, while there is a greater
prevalence of cerebral pathology in the mentally retarded population, the presence of such is not invariably found in all individuals. Figure 1 portrays how the two variables, intelligence
and "brain damage," are distributed in the population. At the low
end of the intelligence distribution there is embedded a brain
pathology distribution, which may or may not be etiologically tied
to the mental retardation of the particular individual.

RELEVANCE OF CLINICAL NEUROPSYCHOLOGY TO MENTAL RETARDATION

From the previous discussion, it is readily apparent that a
substantial percentage of mentally retarded individuals have cerebral pathology. Whether these individuals differ from those without detectable pathology is of major concern. Numerous theoretical discussions and literature reviews have already addressed
this issue (Das, 1972; Ellis, 1969; Weisz & Zigler, 1979; Zigler,
1967; 1969; 1973).

Clinical neuropsychology, because it is simultaneously descriptive and causally oriented, can help in the determination of
the presence or absence of cerebral pathology. For example, it
can be useful for describing the functional capacities of the
familial retarded, and additionally is capable of elucidating the

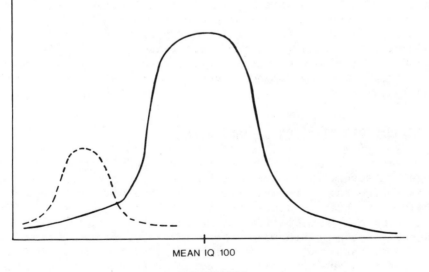

MEAN IQ 100

IQ. DISTRIBUTION

Fig. 1.   The distribution of intelligence and brain damage in the
          normal population.

presence, pattern and extent of cerebral dysfunction for the "organic" conditions. Through multivariate behavioral assessment, neuropsychological measurement can improve our understanding of the various behavioral sequelae that arise from different types of neurological disturbances (Hecaen & Albert, 1978; Reitan & Davidson, 1974). Moreover, neuropsychological techniques afford the opportunity to determine how psychological processes are functionally organized in the brain (Walsh, 1978). Finally, in cases where the etiology is unknown, neuropsychological procedures can help determine if subaverage intellectual functioning is a consequence of either focal or diffuse brain pathology. Hence, neuropsychological procedures can assist in differential diagnosis where the presence, pattern and severity of central nervous system dysfunction needs to be clarified.

Because neuropsychological techniques interrelate brain functioning and behavior, the information accrued has both descriptive and explanatory power. As such, it is feasible to generate heuristic etiological hypotheses that could comprise a basis for the development of a comprehensive classification system incorporating both neurological and psychological information. In addition, since the brain is the organ most responsible for mediating communication with the organism's other biological systems, as well as the external environment, it is the final link in determining adaptive capacity. Through extensive functional assessment of behavioral processes (e.g., language, memory, spatial-constructional skills, etc.), that are known to be subserved by specific cerebral regions and systems, it is possible, therefore, to determine both the level and style of the individual's transaction with his social environment. In this regard, it is not surprising, therefore, that neuropsychological measures are predictive of social, vocational, and educational success (Heaton & Pendleton, 1981; Heaton, Chelune, & Lehman, 1978). For these reasons, neuropsychological techniques can not only delineate current functional status, but also the potential adaptive success of mentally retarded individuals.

FUNCTIONAL ORGANIZATION OF THE BRAIN

Neuropsychology makes inferences regarding the status of the neural substrate by observing behavior under standardized conditions. Two basic research strategies have been employed. First, studies have been conducted in which the neural substrate, either by electrical stimulation or surgical ablation, was manipulated, and the effects on behavior recorded. The second strategy has involved examining patients with verified neurological pathology and measuring the changes in behavior. After more than a century of clinical and research investigations employing these two strategies, it is now known in general terms how psychological functions are organized in the brain. These findings are succinctly reviewed below.

Lateralization

The two cerebral hemispheres are structurally and functionally asymmetrical. Normally, in a right handed individual, the left cerebral hemisphere is considered the "dominant hemisphere," because it subserves language processes. The right cerebral hemisphere, on the other hand, typically subserves nonverbal cognitive processes such as visuospatial information processing. A variety of psychological processes summarized in Table 3 below have been found to be differentially lateralized to either the left or right hemisphere (Berent, 1981), although it should be pointed out that there appears to be some degree of bilateral representation of these various processes in both hemispheres.

Table 3. Various functions ascribed to the left and right cerebral hemispheres by various authors

Left Hemisphere	Right Hemisphere
Speech	Spatial Orientation
Language	Picture and Pattern
Complex Motor Functions	Sense
Vigilance	Performance Functions
Paired Associate Learning	Spatial Integration
Liaison to Consciousness	Creative Associative
Verbal Abilities	Thinking
Linguistic Description	Calculation
Ideation	Simple Language
Conceptual Similarities	Comprehension
Analysis Over Time	Nonverbal Ideation
Analysis of Detail	Facial Identification
Arithmetic	Recognition of Common
Writing	Environmental Sounds
Calculation	Nonverbal Paired
Main Language Center	Associate
Finger Naming	Learning
Right-Left Orientation	Tactile Perception

Localization

Within each hemisphere, there is also regional specialization of psychological functions. Figure 2 illustrates the basic divisions of the cortex. Below, each cortical region is discussed with reference to the specific function it subserves. It should

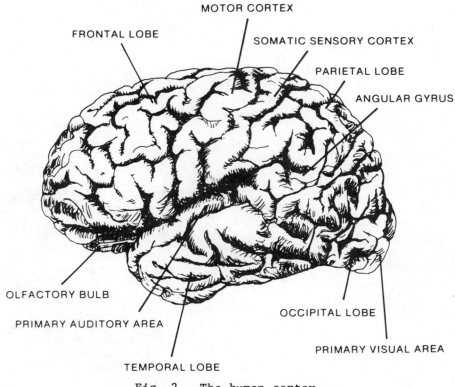

MOTOR CORTEX

FRONTAL LOBE

SOMATIC SENSORY CORTEX

PARIETAL LOBE

ANGULAR GYRUS

OLFACTORY BULB

PRIMARY AUDITORY AREA

OCCIPITAL LOBE

PRIMARY VISUAL AREA

TEMPORAL LOBE

Fig. 2. The human cortex.

be borne in mind, however, that while each of the regions subserve a predominant role, it is through particular neuronal systems and, indeed, the brain as an integral entity, that behavior is effected.

Frontal lobes. This region of the brain has been extensively studied, but yet still remains very much of an enigma. Primary functions subserved by the frontal lobes are the integration of complex motor functions and, in some respects, the mediation of cognitive processes and emotive behavior. Its mode of functioning has been likened very much to that of a computer by serving as a mediator in the processing of information from the external and internal environments. The so-called "executive" functions; that is, the planning, organizing and implementing of behavioral programs, are subserved by the frontal region. Damage to the posterior frontal region of the brain typically results in motor impairments, while a lesion in the anterior frontal area often results in deficits in solving complex problems, behavioral perseverations, reduced cognitive flexibility and incapacity to benefit from feedback in modulating behavior.

Parietal lobes. The sensory strip and association areas of the parietal lobes subserve elementary forms of sensation, as well as praxis and visuospatial capacities. Damage to this cortical area also commonly produces impairments in the ability to recognize modality specific stimuli. These impairments are referred to as *agnosias,* since they result in an incapacity to recognize symbols or objects while leaving the perceptual apparatus intact. For example, the inability to recognize the shapes of objects upon manual manipulation is a tactile agnosia.

Occipital lobes. This brain region, containing the primary visual cortex, is located in the most posterior aspect of the brain. The processing of visual information and symbols, as well as certain visual memory processes, are subserved by this cortical region. Damage in this area of the brain region often results in "scotomas," or "holes" in the visual field, loss of portions of the visual fields, or cortical blindness.

Temporal lobes. This brain region contains the primary sensory regions for audition, and to a lesser extent, olfaction. The temporal lobes play a central role in language processes, and are also integral for memory functioning. One of the most enigmatic functions of the temporal lobes relates to the mediation of emotion through associations with underlying subcortical and limbic structures. For example, partial complex seizures often have their lesion locus in the temporal lobes, and frequently result in intense expression of emotionality and bizarre behavior, as well as dissociative states of consciousness. Damage to the temporal lobes, as with other cortical regions, produces disturbances that depend on the lateralization of the insult. Lesions in the right temporal lobe, for example, can result in a variety of disturbances in essentially nonverbal auditory and memory functions, while lesions in the left temporal lobe tend to result in disruption of receptive and repetitive language processes.

This very brief overview of cerebral lateralization and regional specialization summarizes the basic features of functional brain organization. The reader is referred to Hecaen and Albert (1978), Walsh (1978), Heilman and Valenstein (1979), Filskov and Boll (1981), and Lezak (1976) for more extensive discussions.

RATIONALE UNDERLYING NEUROPSYCHOLOGICAL ASSESSMENT PROCEDURES

The primary goals of a neuropsychological assessment are to: 1) provide a description of the current behavioral or functional status of the individual presumed to be brain damaged; 2) identify, where possible, underlying etiology; and, 3) develop recommendations for treatment that are specific to the nature and extent of the identified impairment.

In terms of the general application of neuropsychology to the assessment of brain functional integrity, the following generalizations can be advanced. The neuropsychological examination is a valuable ancillary procedure that complements neurological and radiological techniques of diagnosis. These procedures are particularly useful where there is subtle neurological dysfunction, such as in many of the developmental disorders that may not be detectable by other means of assessment. The neuropsychological evaluation can thus increase the discriminative capacity of the overall neurodiagnostic process.

A neuropsychological evaluation can also yield important information about level of functioning that can be subsequently monitored over time or during the course of treatment. This enables interventions that could accelerate the recovery of function, or prevent further deterioration of function as in the case of the progressive neuropathies. Such data generating capacity, when combined with knowledge of the clinical course or typical style of recovery from certain forms of brain injury, further allows prognostic inferences about the future behavioral status the patient is likely to attain.

Once the comprehensive diagnostic process is completed, the neuropsychologist can advise on and implement treatment interventions. By detailing the person's adaptive strengths and limitations, interventions can be developed that are targeted to specific functional impairments.

By applying neuropsychological procedures, similar benefits to the mentally retarded individual can be accrued. At the descriptive level, neuropsychological procedures can assist in the delineation of the specific characteristics of the various mental retardation syndromes. To the extent that neuropsychological measurements tap a wider range of cognitive functions than revealed by the mental age or intelligence quotient, and also have an anatomical referent, they surpass psychometric tests of intelligence. Consequently, a more diverse and comprehensive pool of information is available upon which to draw inferences or hypotheses regarding cerebral integrity. In addition, it is possible to itemize general strengths and weaknesses across a broad range of cognitive and behavioral processes. This specificity of measurement is particularly important where deficits are circumscribed to a particular modality. Hence, the neuropsychological examination can determine the level, range and specificity of cerebral pathology, measured in functional terms, that can provide a basis for habilitation.

In addition, a neuropsychological assessment of the mentally retarded person can provide a more valid perspective of functional capacity than is possible with psychometric tests of intelligence. Indeed, the latter measures may even present a biased or distorted picture of psychological impairment. For instance, a child suffering from cerebral palsy, by virtue of the neuromotor disability, performs poorly on timed tests that require motor dexterity. This noncognitive deficit would inevitably result in a lowered IQ score on the Wechsler Performance Scales, thereby opening the way for misclassification, or at best confounded data. Similarly, a child of normal intelligence suffering from an attention deficit disorder generally performs poorly on tests that require sustained concentration or vigilance. The ensuing low summary IQ score could also result in a misdiagnosis. Neuropsychological procedures afford the opportunity to identify and separate the factors responsible for impaired capacity. Thus, while psychometric tests may reveal a low IQ, neuropsychological procedures can relate this to specific perceptual, attentional, memory, language, or motor processes. Hence, not only will diagnosis be more accurate, but the treatment to follow will also be more appropriate.

THE METHODOLOGY OF NEUROPSYCHOLOGICAL ASSESSMENT

Two basic strategies have traditionally been employed in neuropsychological assessment. These are the quantitative and qualitative approaches to describing behavior.

Adherents to the quantitative approach argue that the focus on the neuropsychological assessment must be on the measurable overt aspects of behavior. In contrast, the qualitative orientation emphasizes the stylistic aspects of performance. An example of the divergent perspectives is illustrated by the way an individual's performance on the Block Design test of the WISC or WAIS is scored or interpreted. The quantitatively oriented examiner evaluates performance based upon an interpretation of the standard score. Hence, a score above or below the population mean score reflects a deviation from the norm in either a positive or negative direction. The qualitatively oriented examiner, on the other hand, approaches the situation by observing the patient's strategy in performing the task, such as how he plans, organizes, and integrates perceptual and motor processes. Thus, the strategy for task execution (e.g., logical versus trial and error) is considered valuable information by the qualitatively oriented neuropsychologist. While there is much controversy surrounding the superiority of one or the other of these two approaches (Goldstein, 1981), it should be emphasized that they need not be considered mutually exclusive. In actual practice, the assessment of the multiply handicapped or severely impaired patient, requires the application of techniques that have been developed from each of these two perspectives. For example, on many occasions, a complete or standardized evaluation is not feasible. Under such circumstances, an experienced clinician may, however, be able to obtain valuable neuropsychological information by combining observational and quantitative data.

Thus, familiarity with both quantitative and qualitative aspects of test administration and interpretation is essential for a comprehensive neuropsychological assessment, especially for cases involving the lower end of the functioning continuum. Depending on the patient's specific needs and capacities, the test battery can include measures that range along a continuum of highly quantitative and objective tests to less structured tasks that enable observation and inference of cognitive style.

The Halstead-Reitan Neuropsychological Test Battery best exemplifies test construction oriented to quantitative measurement (Reitan, 1979). The patient is administered a battery of cognitive, motor, and perceptual tests, along with the WAIS or WISC. An "impairment index," having a range of zero to one, is obtained which describes the likelihood and severity of cerebral pathology. Depending on the particular pattern among the various measures, it is also possible to accurately infer lesion localization and lateralization. The battery can be administered in three forms, depending on the age of the person, with the earliest applicable age being for elementary school age children. For a more thorough coverage of the Halstead-Reitan Battery, the reader is referred to Boll (1978, 1981) and Golden (1979).

Luria (1973, 1980) perhaps best represents the quintessential characteristics of the qualitatively oriented neuropsychologist. The examination, as conducted by Luria, is not standardized. An advantage of this is that it allows for flexibility in testing hypotheses about the underlying causes for the behavioral deficits. However, Luria's methodology requires a fund of knowledge and experience that far surpasses that possessed by the average clinician. Another limitation is that his methods do not readily lend themselves to empiricial investigation. Golden, Hammeke, and Purisch (1978), cognizant of these problems, developed a standardized battery that attempted to preserve the qualitative inferential power of the conceptualization, but at the same time also to yield standardized and quantitative information and, hence, to attend to the important issues of test validity and reliability. The Luria-Nebraska Neuropsychological Battery, the product of this effort, thus enables the opportunity to observe the patient perform multiple cognitive operations, but additionally contains fourteen separate scales that can be profiled in a format similar to an MMPI profile. Both adult and children versions of the battery are available. Excellent reviews of this battery can be found in Golden (1981a,b), and a more critical discussion of its theoretical basis and validity can be found in Lezak (1982).

Because no single test of cerebral pathology is sufficient for valid differential diagnosis, a number of different batteries and combinations of tests have been proposed. They can be grouped into two basic types: a) the "screening battery," and, b) the "extended battery." If the question is only to determine if a patient is either neurologically impaired or not, the screening battery will generally suffice. For example, in a community mental health facility, where large numbers of patients are assessed daily, a relatively short, but efficient, battery is desirable in order to first detect patients who are cerebrally impaired, and for whom further extensive evaluation is then warranted. Under these circumstances, several tests that have "cutting-score" criteria; that is, ability to correctly classify the individual as cognitively impaired at an empirically ascertained level of statistical certainty, will generally suffice.

Screening batteries typically reflect the biases and objectives of the particular neuropsychologist. Usually, tests that are brief but yet sufficiently discriminative, are incorporated into a battery. Golden (1979), for example, suggests a screening battery composed of four WAIS subtests (Object Assembly, Block Design, Similarities, and Digit Symbol) along with the Stroop Color Word Test, the Speech Perception Rhythm Test, and the Aphasia Test. This combination of tests is claimed to identify the presence of cerebral pathology with approximately 90% accuracy, while taking only ninety minutes to administer. Goldstein, Tarter, Shelly and Hegdus (1984) have proposed a screening battery which measures intelligence and level of performance, as well as language, memory, motor and spatial-constructional processes. A unique feature of the battery is the availability of computerized age correction of the raw data into a profile. The examiner is thus provided with a readily utilizable format for interpretation of the data. The advantage of this procedure is that comparisons can be made between the different areas of neuropsychological functioning. The total test time is about ninety minutes, and the battery can be administered to individuals as young as thirteen years of age.

The screening battery in general, due to its limited breadth of processes measured, is often not sufficient for clinical decision making in retarded populations. Frequently, the mentally retarded patient may appear as globally impaired due to their presenting intellectual incapacity. Therefore, a broader range of measures may be required in order to detect particular areas of strength and weakness within the total context of mental retardation.

When a more comprehensive description of deficits associated with cerebral dysfunction is required, the neuropsychologist can draw upon a rather large armamentarium of test measures. The more commonly used tests which are applicable to retarded populations are listed in the Appendix at the end of this chapter. In addition to the children's form of the Halstead-Reitan and Luria-Nebraska batteries, there are numerous tests which can be accessed to evaluate virtually all aspects of functional or adaptive capacity. Lezak (1983) provides a description of many of these measures.

The utilization of a comprehensive standardized battery has certain advantages over screening procedures. First, the examiner can employ the battery knowing that reliability and validity criteria have been met. Second, comprehensive batteries provide a common referrent for the conduct of research in clinical neuropsychology, thus permitting comparability of test findings between investigators and across populations. There are, however, also certain limitations in the utilization of comprehensive batteries. Duration of testing time is one major consideration. The relative worth of an extensive examination must be determined on the basis of the value of the information to be derived, as well as the capacity of the patient to participate in this type of evaluation. In severely impaired patients, alternative forms of assessment may be necessary. In addition, the breadth of functions covered by a comprehensive assessment is achieved at the expense of diminished depth, a factor which is of concern where subtle deficits may be present. The variety of behavioral manifestations of cerebral pathology are such that all potential areas of investigation cannot be covered by a single inflexible battery.

One strategy aimed at avoiding the above limitations is to use an assessment protocol that is tailored to the particular

needs of each patient. Through a continuous and ongoing process
of hypothesis testing by the examiner, the evaluation can be conducted so as to answer as many questions as possible. The work of
Luria (1966) exemplifies this approach and the plethora of tests
described by Lezak (1983) and described in the Appendix to this
chapter illustrate the potential value of conducting assessments
in this fashion. It should be pointed out, however, that while
this clinical approach offers both flexibility and comprehensive-
ness, it does not enable the examiner to establish a coherent
database, either for research purposes, or to readily conduct
clinical outcome investigations.

INTERPRETATION OF NEUROPSYCHOLOGICAL TEST DATA

Lezak (1976) notes that a neuropsychological assessment is
quite similar to a conventional psychological examination. In the
routine psychological evaluation, the examiner focuses upon the
patient's intellectual status, personality characteristics and
emotional state. Situational and historical factors, as well as
coping style and adjustment success, are also evaluated where
possible. From this pool of information, a diagnostic impression
is derived and recommendations regarding treatment are proposed.
The neuropsychological examination proceeds essentially along the
same lines, but with an emphasis upon the person's "deficits,'
particularly inasmuch as they are attributable to cerebral pathology.

In mental retardation, as in other types of disorders, three
types of test based information are obtained. These pertain to:
a) pathognomonic signs; b) cutting scores; and, c) pattern analysis.

Pathognomonic Signs

The sign approach is based upon the premise that there are
distinct characteristics or manifestations of brain damage that
can be reliably and validly identified. Typically, these "signs"
pertain to behaviors which are readily observable during the testing, or in the patient's natural environment. Sattler (1982) provides a detailed description of the range of pathognomonic signs
that might be revealed by a neuropsychological examination of
which a summary can be found in Table 4.

Cutting Scores

These scores differentiate brain damaged from non-brain
damaged individuals on the basis of criterion scores. Cutting
scores are most commonly utilized in screening batteries. While
the possibility of misclassification is inherently problematic in
this approach, employing cutting scores has, nonetheless, proven

Table 4.   Possible signs and symptoms of brain damage observed on the neuropsychological examination

Area	Sign or Symptom
Motor	Hyperkinesis (constant movement, inability to sit still; fingering, touching, and mouthing objects; voluble and uninhibited speech); awkwardness in locomotion (clumsiness, atypical arm swing, incoordination, tremors, involuntary movements, asymmetry of facial musculature and expressive gestures while talking); awkwardness in skilled movement (poor printing, writing, and drawing); impaired copying of geometric designs; postural rigidity; speech difficulties (e.g., dysarthria, slow speech); mixed dominance, repetitive movements; and perseveration
Sensory	Short attention span; poor concentration; distractibility; perceptual difficulty (e.g., closure difficulty, visual-motor disturbances, use of fingers to guide movements, turning materials around); and unusual episodic sensory experiences (e.g., occurrence of odd odors or vision of lights)
Affective	Reduced frustration threshold; emotional lability (impulsivity, irritability, aggressiveness, easily moved to tears, loss of control of emotions); anxiety (occasional panic reactions); and depression
Cognitive	Some intellectual deficit; impaired judgement; conceptual difficulties (e.g., in abstracting, planning, organizing, anticipating, analyzing and synthesizing, and integrating); specific learning deficit (in reading, spelling, or arithmetic); language difficulties (e.g., malapropisms, imprecise synonyms, truncated sentences, mispronunciations, circumstantiality); attraction to minute details; impaired right-left orientation; perseveration; concrete, rigid, and inflexible thinking; difficulty in shifting; and memory difficulty (recent, remote, or both, visual, auditory, or both)
Social	Interpersonal difficulties; immaturity (e.g., may regress to more childlike forms of behavior); negativism; and antisocial behavior (lying, stealing, truancy, sexual offenses)
Personality	Disturbed self-concept; disturbed body concept or body image; changes in personality (e.g., a previ-

ously fastidious child becomes unkempt and care-
less); hypochondriacal preoccupations; compulsive
tendencies; denial (e.g., children may deny that
they have any problems); and indications of
insecurity (e.g., expressions of weakness, uncer-
tainty, and inadequacy in dealing with test materials)

From Jerome M. Sattler, ASSESSMENT OF CHILDREN'S INTELLIGENCE AND
SPECIAL ABILITIES, 2nd Edition. Copyright © 1982 by Allyn and
Bacon, Inc. Reprinted with permission.

to be highly capable of differentiating brain damaged from normal
individuals.

Pattern Analysis

This procedure allows for easy interpretation of both intra-
test scatter (variability of performance within a subtest), and
inter-test scatter (variability between subtests). Pattern analysis is particularly useful where different tests and functions are
described along a common scale. An example is the previously discussed Pittsburgh Initial Neuropsychological Test System (Goldstein et al., 1984), where numerous measures are transformed into
a T-scale for easy comparison. Pattern analysis remains very much
an "art," and thus depends on the clinical accumen and experience
of the examiner. However, several statistical programs have been
developed, and are discussed by Rourke and Adams in this volume.

NEUROPSYCHOLOGICAL ASSESSMENT OF THE MENTALLY RETARDED

The primary objective of a neuropsychological evaluation is
to delineate the patient's cognitive and behavioral strengths and
limitations. Inferences about the location and type of the underlying cerebral lesion are secondary considerations.

The evaluation process begins, where possible, with a
detailed developmental history. The reader is referred to Gardner
(1979) for a concise parent questionnaire that details the child's
developmental history. Reports of recent physical examinations,
neurological consultations, and prior psychological assessments
are very helpful at the outset in defining the problem and objectives of the neuropsychological evaluation. Educational records
should also be obtained since they provide information about base-
line levels of functioning, and document any changes in cognitive
performances that have taken place.

Prior to the neuropsychological assessment, it is recommended
that intelligence testing be conducted. Where intellectual

capacity is severely limited, the Stanford Binet Form L-M (Terman & Merrill, 1960) is preferred over the WISC-R (Wechsler, 1974), inasmuch as it taps cognitive functions at a basal level lower than that assessed on the Wechsler Scales. The utilization of a "Binetgram" (Sattler, 1965) provides the examiner with a profile of cognitive functions. The psychological functions described in the profile, though not originally intended for neuropsychological interpretation, can nonetheless be used for these purposes. The McCarthy Scales (McCarthy, 1970), are another alternative to the WISC-R and have the advantage of Memory and Motor subtests in addition to Verbal, Performance, and Full Scale IQ indices.

There are at least two reasons to begin the neuropsychological evaluation with an intelligence assessment. First, it affords the opportunity to observe qualitative aspects of performance by inspecting profile patterns (e.g., discrepancy between Verbal IQ and Performance IQ) which could subsequently facilitate the formulation of neuropsychological hypotheses. Second, performance on tests of intelligence may itself constitute an index of cerebral pathology. Sattler (1982) contains an excellent discussion of specific pathognomonic signs of cerebral pathology that can be accrued from the WISC-R and Stanford Binet Form L-M.

Along with a neuropsychological investigation, the patient should also be assessed for current level of academic achievement. Information obtained from this type of evaluation not only describes current educational status, but also serves as a reference point to relate past and future academic functioning. By directly comparing IQ and current level of academic performance, it can be determined if the patient is functioning above, below, or within a reasonable range of expectation for his intellectual capacity. This type of information is particularly important for determining the rate of change of a specific cerebral condition. In addition, educational measures may provide heuristic hypotheses about the locus of a lesion. For example, a parietal-occipital lesion would be suspect if there is a circumscribed reading and spelling deficit. Within the context of general intellectual impairment, it is not unusual for a circumscribed neuropsychological impairment to also exist (Benton, 1970). Finally, academic achievement testing is critical in situations where the differential diagnosis of specific learning disability versus mental retardation is an issue. Boder (1973), for example, stresses the importance of accurate differential diagnosis of reading retardation in the mentally retarded. She notes that developmental dyslexia, as a syndrome separate and distinct from generalized or nonspecific reading retardation, can indeed coexist with mental retardation. In order to develop adequate and appropriate remedial intervention, differential diagnostic assessment becomes especially critical. Measures such as the Wide Range Achievement Test (Jastak & Jastak, 1965), the Peabody Individual Achievement

Test (Dunn & Markwardt, 1970), and the Detroit Test of Learning
Aptitude (DTLA) (Baker & Leland, 1967), are some of the more
commonly employed tests of academic achievement.

Another important component of the evaluation process for
mental retardation concerns delineating adaptive sociobehavioral
capacities. Several instruments are available, all of which have
approximately equal utility. The AAMD Adaptive Behavior Scale,
because of its graphic representation of ten behavior domains,
though not the most comprehensive, is one of the most commonly
utilized instruments (Nihira et al., 1974). For very low level
functioning patients, the Balthazar Scales of Adaptive Behavior
may, however, provide more pertinent information (Balthazar,
1971).

Finally, as part of a comprehensive neuropsychological evaluation of mentally retarded persons, it is necessary to assess
emotional status. Personality assessment of retardates often,
however, necessitates, for obvious reasons, modifications of
instruments originally designed for use in the general population. Karp et al. (1978) describes tests like the Rorschach,
Thematic Apperception Test, and Figure Drawing which can be
adapted for use with the retarded population. Certain standardized personality inventories, such as the MMPI, particularly in an
abbreviated form, if orally administered, can reveal important
information about concurrent psychopathology and personality dis-
position. Because brain damage increases the risk for a psychiatric disorder (Rutter, 1977), this component of the evaluation
process should not, if at all possible, be overlooked.

These four components, consisting of intellectual, educational, social adaptive and psychopathological-personality variables,
provide the clinician with a substantial inventory of data and
observational material that broadens the coverage of the assessment and increases the validity of the interpretation. The comprehensive neuropsychological evaluation, using the above information as a backdrop, will additionally evaluate the following
dimensions of psychological functioning: 1) general level of performance; 2) conceptual or abstracting ability; 3) sensory functions; 4) perceptual capacity; 5) memory; 6) language; 7) motor
ability; 8) visuospatial capacities; and, 9) constructional abilities. Specific tests that are available and commonly used to
measure these neuropsychological processes are described in the
Appendix to the chapter.

Where a focal lesion is suspected, additional considerations
must also be given to the following factors in selecting a test
battery and interpreting the various scores.
    1) the site of the lesion.
    2) the size, severity and course of the lesion process.

3) the likely causal agent(s).
4) the patient's age at the time the lesion occurred.
5) the premorbid status of the patient.
6) the length of time between the onset of the sus-
    tained damage and the date of actual testing.
7) the general physical status and health of the
    patient.
8) the quality of the environmental support system.

All of the above factors influence neuropsychological performance and should be addressed in interpreting a particular profile
of scores. With respect to mental retardation, this process may
be especially difficult since etiology may either be not identifiable or multifactorial in nature. Also, more often than not,
there is no circumscribed lesion. Furthermore, the empirical substrate upon which clinical neuropsychology rests, is essentially
based on studies conducted on brain damaged adults. The generalizations that can be drawn from adults to children where the brain
is still developing, are thus tenuous. Moreover, little direct
research of the applicability and validity of applying neuropsychological measures to th- ˙ ˛'or ˛ ˙ ˀ˙ abilities has been
conducted. Even though there is a convincing rationale for conducting neuropsychological research and clinical evaluations in
mental retardation, the application of these procedures has been
surprisingly limited. Considering, however, the number of individuals in society with mental retardation, and the value of the
information contained in a neuropsychological assessment, a more
concerned effort to use these procedures would appear to be
strongly warranted (Benton, 1970; Gordon, 1977; Baumeister, &
MacLean, 1979; Tarter, & Slomka, 1983).

APPENDIX

A brief description of the major areas assessed in a clinical
neurological evaluation is presented below. Within each category,
several tests, or components of tests, that are applicable to the
assessment of the mentally retarded are listed. The reader is
referred to Buros (1978), Lezak (1976), Gardner (1979), and
Herbert (1964) for more detailed descriptions of the various
instruments.

Level of Performance

Tests subsumed within this category measure how well or
poorly a person performs a specific task. These tests can identify the presence of cerebral pathology, but are not sensitive to
localizing or lateralizing a lesion. Basically, poor performance
on these tests reflects decremental functioning associated with
most forms of cerebral pathology. The following are examples of
tests of general performance level.

Symbol-Digit Modalities Test (Smith, 1976)
Trail Making Test (Reitan, 1958, 1979)
Stroop Color-Word Test (Dodrill, 1978)
Purdue Pegboard (Tifflin, 1968)

The level of performance concept can also be applied to measures of intellectual functioning. The *g* factor in intelligence,
although disputed by some, is nonetheless an index of general
intellect and capacity. Somewhat more specific, but still
anchored empirically to broad aspects of intellectual functioning,
are the verbal and performance subscale IQ scores of the Wechsler
scales. These, as well as other measures, yield general indices
of overall cognitive level, a psychological construct that is not
amenable to cerebral localization. Tests of cognitive or intellectual capacity that are applicable to the mentally retarded
include:

Wechsler Intelligence Scales for children and adults
    (Wechsler, 1955, 1974)
Stanford Binet Form L-M (Terman & Merrill, 1960)
McCarthy Scales of Children's Abilities (McCarthy, 1970)
Arthur Point Scale of Performance Tests (Arthur, 1947)
Peabody Picture Vocabulary Test (Dunn, 1965)
Ravens Progressive Matrices (Raven, 1960)
Leiter International Performance Scale (Leiter, 1959)
Pictorial Test of Intelligence (French, 1964)

Conceptual Ability

Brain damage often results in a diminished capacity to
appreciate the relationships between objects and their properties. An impairment in abstract thinking can occur in association
with pathology anywhere in the cerebrum, although usually this
deficit is evident in cases of diffuse lesions. The following
tests are measures of abstracting or conceptual ability:

Similarities subtest of the WAIS (Wechsler, 1955)
Object Sorting Test (Goldstein & Scheerer, 1941)
The Category Test (Reitan, 1979)
Proverbs Test (Gorham, 1956)

Perceptual and Sensory Capacities

Lezak (1976) distinguishes two levels of perceptual analysis: 1) sensory reception in the visual, auditory, tactile, and
kinesthetic modalities; and, 2) sensory input that is organized
and integrated into psychologically meaningful information in the
form of perceptions. A cerebral lesion can result in the loss of
a specific sensory modality (e.g., blindness, deafness), or produce an agnosia; that is, the total or partial loss of the ability
to discriminate, recognize, organize or structure sensory input

into its knowable form. Where sensory impairment is suspected, the following tests are suggested:

>Screening Test for Auditory Acuity (Bolies, 1954)
>Formal Audiometric Examination
>Schrier Visual Screening Test (Gardner, 1979)
>Sensory-Perceptual Examination of the Halstead Reitan Battery (Reitan, 1979)

Perceptual functions can be assessed using the following tests:

>Illinois Test of Psycholinguistic Ability (Kirk, McCarthy & Kirk, 1968)
>Boston Diagnostic Aphasia Examination (Goodglass & Kaplan, 1976)
>Rhythm Test (Reitan, 1979)
>Speech Sounds Perception Test (Reitan, 1979)
>Token Test (Boller & Dennis, 1979)
>Hooper Visual Organization Test (Hooper, 1958)
>Maze Tests of WISC and Stanford Binet (Wechsler, 1974; Terman & Merrill, 1960)
>Ravens Progressive Matrices (Raven, 1960)
>Developmental Test of Visual Perception (Frostig et al., 1966)
>Frostig
>Developmental Test of Visuomotor Integration (Beery, 1967)
>Tactile Performance Test (Reitan, 1979)

Memory

Efficacy of learning and memory is frequently diminished in persons with cerebral pathology. Memory can be variously assessed and should include measures of short- and long-term recall, as well as evaluations of modality specific information. Several of the common tests of memory are:

>Wechsler Memory Scale (Wechsler, 1945)
>Memory Subtests of the McCarthy Scale (McCarthy, 1970)
>Memory Subtests of the Stanford Binet form L-M (Terman & Merrill, 1960)
>Digit Span Tests (various forms): (Wechsler, 1955, 1974; Terman & Merrill, 1960), as well as a nonverbal administration, the Point Digit Span
>Sound Blending and Auditory Closure (Kirk et al., 1968)
>Berkley Paired Associate Learning Test (Lambert et al., 1974)
>Visual Sequential Memory (Kirk et al., 1968)
>Benton Revised Visual Retention Test (Benton, 1963)
>Graham-Kendall Memory for Designs Test (Graham & Kendall, 1960)
>Tactual Performance Test (Reitan, 1979) (Baker & Leland, 1967)
>Detroit Test of Learning Aptitude

Special consideration must be given to attentional capacities since an impairment in these processes could affect memory. Several measures can be employed to evaluate attentional ability:

> Digit Span, Coding, Mazes, Arithmetic Subtests of the WISC-R (Wechsler, 1968)
> Visual Closure Test of the ITPA (Kirk et al., 1968)
> Klove-Knights Steadiness Test (Knights, 1966)
> Symbol Digit Modalities Test (Smith, 1976)
> Trailmaking Test (Reitan, 1958)

Language

Language capacities of the mentally retarded can be assessed to determine the general level of maturational development, as well as to evaluate whether there are specific impairments that are localizable in the cortex.

> Boston Diagnostic Aphasia Examination (Goodglass & Kaplan, 1972)
> Aphasia Screening Test (Russell, Neuringer, & Goldstein, 1970)
> Token Test (Boller & Dennis, 1979)
> Modification of the Halstead-Wepman Aphasia Screening Test (Reitan, 1979)
> Illinois Test of Psycholinguistic Abilities (Kirk et al., 1968)
> Peabody Picture Vocabulary Test (Dunn, 1965)
> Expressive One-Word Vocabulary Test

Motor Capacity

Boll and Barth (1981) distinguish three types of tests of motor capacities: 1) tests of speed, strength, coordination; 2) tests of motor persistence; and, 3) tests of motor steadiness. Assessment of motor integrity in the mentally retarded has significant habilitation implications, inasmuch as it bears on the retardates' capacity to physically relate to the environment. The following tests are frequently used to measure motor capacity:

> Finger Oscillation Test or Finger Tapping Test; a component of the Halstead-Reitan Battery (Halstead, 1947; Reitan & Davison, 1974)
> Strength of Grip Test (Reitan, 1979)
> Tactile Performance Tests (Reitan, 1979)
> Purdue Pegboard Test (Lafayette Instrument Co.)
> Brunincks-Oseretsky Test of Motor Proficiency
> Finger-Thumb Opposition (Denckla, 1973, 1974)
> Mazes (WISC-R, subtest) (Wechsler, 1974)
> Tests of Motor Impersistence (Garfield, 1964)
> Steadiness Test (Gardner, Craemmerer, & Broman, 1979)
> Southern California Sensory Integration Tests (Ayres, 1972)

Visuospatial and Constructional Capacity

These processes involve the ability to reproduce geometric designs, or perform three dimensional constructions:

Bender Gestalt Test (Bender, 1938)
Minnesota Percepto-Diagnostic Test (Fuller, 1969)
Rey-Osterreith Complex Figure Test (Lezak, 1976)
Benton Visual Retention Test: Copy Administration (Benton, 1963)
Memory for Designs Test (Graham & Kendall, 1960)
Aphasia Screening Test (Russell et al., 1970)
Block Design and Object Assembly of WISC-R (Wechsler, 1955, 1974)
Stick Test (Butters & Barton, 1970)
Paper Folding: Triangle Level V Stanford Binet (Terman & Merrill, 1960)

REFERENCES

Arthur, G. **A point scale of performance tests.** (rev. 2nd ed.). New York: Macmillan, 1972.

Ayres, J. **Southern California Sensory Integration Tests.** Los Angeles: Western Psychological Services, 1972.

Baker, H. & Leland, B. **Detroit Tests of Learning Aptitude. Examiners handbook.** Indianapolis, IN, 1967.

Balthazar, E. **Balthazar Scales of Adaptive Behavior.** Palo Alto, CA: Consulting Psychologists Press, Inc., 1971.

Baumeister, A. & MacLean, W. Brain damage and mental retardation. In N. Ellis (Ed.), **Handbook of mental deficiency: Psychological theory and research.** Hillsdale, NJ: Lawrence Erlbaum, 1979.

Beery, K. **Developmental Test of Visual-motor Integration.** Chicago: Follett Publishing Co., 1967.

Bender, L. A visual motor gestalt test and its clinical use. **American Orthopsychiatric Association Research Monographs,** no. 3, 1938.

Benton, A.L. **The Revised Visual Retention Test: clinical and experimental applications.** New York: Psychological Corporation, 1963.

Benton, A.L. Neuropsychological aspects of mental retardation. **Journal of Special Education,** 1970, 4, 3–11.

Berent, S. Lateralization of brain function. In S. Filskov & T. Boll, (Eds.), **Handbook of clinical neuropsychology.** New York: John Wiley and Sons, 1981.

Berg, E. A simple objective test for measuring flexibility in thinking. **Journal of General Psychology,** 1948, 39, 15–22.

Boder, E. Developmental dyslexia: A diagnostic approach based on three atypical reading-spelling patterns. **Developmental Medicine and Child Neurology,** 1973, 15, 633–687.

Boles, L. **Fundamentals of otolaryngology.** Philadelphia: W. B. Saunders Co., 1954.

Boll, T.J. Diagnosing brain impairment. In B. Wolman (Ed.), **Clinical diagnosis of mental disorders: A handbook.** New York: Plenum, 1978.

Boll, T.J. The Halstead-Reitan Neuropsychological Battery. In S. Filskov & T. Boll (Eds.), **Handbook of clinical neuropsychology.** New York: John Wiley and Sons, 1981.

Boll, T.J. & Barth, J.T. Neuropsychology of brain damage in children. In S. Filskov & T. Boll: **Handbook of clinical neuropsychology.** New York: John Wiley and Sons, 1981.

Boller, F. & Dennis, M. **Auditory comprehension: Clinical and experimental studies with the Token Test.** New York: Academic Press, 1979.

Bruininks, R. **Bruininks-Oseretsky Test of Motor Proficiency.** Circle Pines, MN: American Guidance Service, 1978.

Buros, O. **The eighth mental measurements yearbook.** Highland Park, NJ: Gryphon Press, 1978.

Butters, N. & Barton, M. Effect of parietal lobe damage on performance of reversible orientations in space. **Neuropsychologia**, 1970, 8, 205-214.

Crome, L. The brain and mental retardation. **British Medical Journal**, 1960, 1, 897-904.

Das, J.P. Patterns of cognitive ability in nonretarded and retarded children. **American Journal of Mental Deficiency**, 1972, 77, 6-12.

Denckla, M. Development of speed in repetitive and successive finger movements in normal children. **Developmental Medicine and Child Neurology**, 1966, 15, 635-645.

Denckla, M. Development of motor coordination in normal children. **Developmental Medicine and Child Neurology**, 1976, 16, 729-741.

Dodrill, C. A neuropsychological battery for epilepsy. **Epilepsia**, 1978, **19**, 611-623.

DSM II: **Diagnostic and statistical manual of mental disorders** (2nd ed.). Washington, DC: American Psychiatric Association, 1968.

DSM III: **Diagnostic and statistical manual of mental disorders**, Washington, DC: American Psychiatric Association, 1980.

Dunn, L.M. **Expanded manual for the Peabody Picture Vocabulary Test.** Circle Pines, MN: American Guidance Service, 1965.

Dunn, L. & Markwardt, F. **Manual. Peabody Individual Achievement Test.** Circle Pines, MN: American Guidance Service, 1970.

Ellis, N.R. A behavioral research strategy in mental retardation: Defense and critique. **American Journal of Mental Deficiency**, 1969, 73, 557-566.

Filskov, S.B. & Boll, T.J. **Handbook of clinical neuropsychology.** New York: John Wiley and Sons, 1981.

French, J.L. **Manual. Pictorial Test of Intelligence.** Boston: Houghton Mifflin, 1964.

Frostig, M., Lefever, W., & Whittlessey, J. **Marianne Frostig Developmental Test of Visual Perception** (Revised manual). Palo Alto, CA: Consulting Psychologists Press, 1966.

Fuller, G. **The Minnesota Percepto-Diagnostic Test** (Rev. ed.). Brandon, VT: Clinical Psychology Publishing Co., 1969.

Gardner, A., Caemmerer, A., & Broman, M. An instrument for measuring hyperactivity and other signs of minimal brain dysfunction. **Journal of Clinical Child Psychology**, 1979, 8, 173–179.

Gardner, R.A. **The objective diagnosis of minimal brain dysfunction.** Cresskill, NJ: Creative Therapeutics, 1979.

Garfield, J. Motor impersistence in normal and brain damaged children. **Neurology**, 1964, 14, 623–630.

Golden, C.J. **Clinical interpretation of objective psychological tests.** New York: Grune and Stratton, 1979.

Golden, C.J. A standardized version of Luria's Neuropsychological Tests. In S. Filskov & T. Boll (Eds.), **Handbook of clinical neuropsychology.** New York: John Wiley and Sons, 1981(a).

Golden, C. The Luria-Nebraska Neuropsychological Battery: Theory and research. In P. McReynolds (Ed.), **Advances in psychological assessment**, Vol. 5. San Francisco: Jossey-Bass, 1981(b).

Golden, C.J., Hammeke, T., & Purisch, A. Diagnostic validity of the Luria neuropsychological battery. **Journal of Consulting and Clinical Psychology**, 1978, 46, 1258–1265.

Goldstein, G. Some recent developments in clinical neuropsychology. **Clinical Psychology Review**, 1981, 245–268.

Goldstein, G., Tarter, R., Shelly, C., & Hegedus, A. PINTS: a neuropsychological screening battery for psychiatric patients. **Journal of Behavioral Assessment**, in press.

Goldstein, K. & Scheerer, M. Abstract and concrete behavior: an experimental study with special tests. **Psychological Monographs**, 1941, 53 (No. 2).

Goodglass, H. & Kaplan, E. **Assessment of aphasia and related disorders.** Philadelphia: Lea and Febiger, 1972.

Gordon, J.E. Neuropsychology and mental retardation. In I. Bialer & M. Sternlicht (Eds.), **The psychology of mental retardation: Issues and approaches.** New York: Psychological Dimensions, Inc., 1977.

Gorham, D. A Proverbs Test for clinical and experimental use. **Psychological Reports, Monograph Supplement**, 1956, 1, 1–12.

Graham, F.K. & Kendall, B.S. Memory for Designs-Tests: Revised general manual. **Perceptual and Motor Skills Monograph, Supplement**, No. 2-VII, 1960, 11, 147–188.

Grossman, H.J. **Manual on terminology and classification in mental retardation.** Washington, DC: American Association on Mental Deficiency, 1977.

Heaton, R. & Pendleton, M. Use of neuropsychological tests to predict adult patients' everyday functioning. **Journal of Consulting and Clinical Psychology**, 1981, **49**, 807–821.

Heaton, R., Chelune, G. & Lehman, R. Using neuropsychological and personality tests to assess the likelihood of patient employment. **Journal of Nervous and Mental Disease**, 1978, **166**, 408–415.

Hecaen, H. & Albert, M. **Human neuropsychology.** New York: John Wiley and Sons, 1978.

Heilman, K. & Valenstein, E. **Clinical neuropsychology.** New York: Oxford University Press, 1979.

Heimburger, R.F. & Reitan, R.M. Easily administered written test for lateralizing brain lesions. **Journal of Neurosurgery,** 1961, **18**, 301–312.

Herbert, M. The concept and testing of brain-damage in children: A review. **Journal of Child Psychology and Psychiatry**, 1964, **5**, 197–216.

Hooper, H. **The Hooper Visual Organization Test. Manual.** Los Angeles: Western Psychological Services, 1958.

Jastak, J. & Jastak, S. **The Wide Range Achievement Test manual.** Wilmington, DE: Guidance Associates, 1965.

Jellinger, J. Neuropathological features of unclassified mental retardation. In J. Cavanaugh (Ed.), **The brain in unclassified mental retardation.** Baltimore: Williams and Wilkins, 1972.

Karp, E., Morgenstern, M., & Michal-Smith, H. Diagnosing mental deficiency. In B. Wolman (Ed.), **Clinical diagnosis of mental disorders: A handbook.** New York: Plenum, 1978.

Kirk, S.A., McCarthy, J.J., & Kirk, W.D. **The Illinois Test of Psycholinguistic Abilities** (Rev. Ed.). Urbana, IL: University of Illinois Press, 1968.

Klove, H. Clinical neuropsychology. In F. Forster (Ed.), **The medical clinics of North America.** New York: Saunders, 1963.

Knights, R. **Normative data on tests for evaluating brain damage in children from 5 to 14 years of age.** Research Bulletin No. 20, Department of Psychology. London, Canada: University of Western Ontario, 1966.

Lambert, N., Wilcox, M., & Gleason, W. **The educationally retarded child.** New York: Grune and Stratton, 1974.

Leiter, R.G. Part I of the manual for the 1948 revision of the Leiter International Performance Scale: Evidence of the reliability and validity of the Leiter tests. **Psychological Service Center Journal**, 1959, 11, 1–72.

Lezak, M. **Neuropsychological assessment** (2nd ed.). New York: Oxford University Press, 1983.

Luria, A.R. **The working brain.** New York: Basic Books, 1973.

Luria, A.R. **Higher cortical functions in man** (2nd ed.). New York: Basic Books, 1980.

Malamud, N. Neuropathology. In H. Stevens & R. Heber (Eds.), **Mental retardation: A review of research.** Chicago: University Press, 1964.

Masland, R.L.   The prevention of mental subnormality.   In R.
    Masland, S. Surason, & T. Gladwin (Eds.), **Mental subnormal-
    ity.** New York: Basic Books, 1958.
Matthews, C.G. & Klove, H.   **Instruction manual for the Adult
    Neuropsychology Test Battery.** Madison, WI: University of
    Wisconsin Medical School, 1964.
McCarthy, D. **McCarthy Scales of Children's Abilities.** New York:
    The Psychological Corporation, 1970.
Nihira, K., Foster, R., Shellhaas, M., & Leland, H. **AAMD Adaptive
    Behavior Scale,** 1974 Revision. Washington, DC: American
    Association on Mental Deficiency, 1974.
Raven, I. **Guide to the standard progressive matrices.** London:
    H.K. Lewis, 1960.
Reitan, R.   Validity of the Trail Making Test as an indicator of
    organic brain damage. **Perceptual and Motor Skills,** 1958, 8,
    271-276.
Reitan, R. **Manual for administration of Neuropsychological Test
    Batteries for Adults and Children.** Tucson, AZ, 1979.
Reitan, R. & Davison, L.   **Clinical neuropsychology: Current
    status and applications.** New York: Winston/Wiley, 1974.
Russell, E., Neuringer, C., & Goldstein, G. **Assessment of brain
    damage.   A neuropsychological key approach.** New York:
    Wiley-Interscience, 1970.
Rutter, M.   Brain damage syndromes in childhood: Concepts and
    findings. **Journal of Child Psychology and Psychiatry,** 1977,
    18, 1-21.
Sattler, J.M.   Analysis of functions of the 1960 Stanford-Binet
    Intelligence Scale. Form L-M. **Journal of Clinical Psychol-
    ogy,** 1965, 21, 173-179.
Sattler, J.M. **Assessment of children's intelligence.** Philadel-
    phia: W.B. Saunders Co., 1974.
Sattler, J.M. **Assessment of children's intelligence and special
    abilities** (2nd ed.). Newton, MA: Allyn and Bacon, Inc.,
    1982.
Smith, A.   Neuropsychological testing in neurological disorders.
    In W. Friedlander (Ed.), **Advances in neurology** (Vol 7). New
    York: Raven Press, 1975.
Smith, A. **Symbol Digit Modalities Test manual.** Los Angeles:
    Western Psychological Services, 1976.
Tarter, R. & Slomka, G.   The neuropsychology of mental retarda-
    tion. In J. Matson & J. Mulick (Eds.), **Comprehensive handbook
    of mental retardation.** New York: Pergamon Press, 1983.
Terman, L. & Merrill, M.   **Stanford-Binet Intelligence Scale.**
    Boston: Houghton Mifflin, 1960.
Tiffin, J. **Purdue Pegboard examiner manual.** Chicago: Science
    Research Associates, Inc., 1968.
Tredgold, R.F. & Soddy, K. **Textbook of mental deficiency.** Bal-
    timore: Williams and Wilkins, 1963.
Walsh, K. **Neuropsychology: A clinical approach.** New York:
    Churchill Livingston, 1978.

Wechsler, D.   A standardized memory scale for clinical use.
     Journal of Psychology, 1945, 19, 87.
Wechsler, D.   **Wechsler Adult Intelligence Scale.** New York: The
     Psychological Corporation, 1955.
Wechsler, D.   **Wechsler Intelligence Scale for Children-Revised.**
     New York: The Psychological Corporation, 1974.
Weisz, J.R.   Cognitive development in retarded and nonretarded
     persons: Piagetian tests of the similar sequence hypothesis.
     Psychological Bulletin, 1979, 86, 831-851.
Zigler, E.   Familial mental retardation: A continuing dilemma.
     Science, 1967, 157, 578-579.
Zigler, E.   Developmental versus difference theories of mental
     retardation and the problems of motivation. **American Journal
     of Mental Deficiency**, 1968, 73, 536-556.
Zigler, E.   The retarded child as a whole person.   In D. Routh
     (Ed.), **The experimental psychology of mental retardation.**
     Chicago, IL: Aldine Publishing Co., 1973.

HEAD INJURIES IN CHILDREN: A MODEL FOR PREDICTING COURSE OF RECOVERY AND PROGNOSIS

Harry Klonoff and David D. Crockett

Department of Psychiatry
Division of Psychology
University of British Columbia
Vancouver, British Columbia

and

Campbell Clark

Department of Nuclear Medicine
National Institute of Health
Bethesda, Maryland

Given the scope of the health problems deriving from head injuries of children, there is a paucity of comprehensive studies and, in particular, insufficient information regarding psychological sequelae. The more relevant published studies during the past decade have included Brink, Garrett, Hale, Woo-Sam, and Nickel (1970), Black, Blumer, Wellner, and Walker (1971), Klonoff (1971), Klonoff and Low (1974), Klonoff and Paris (1974), Mandleberg and Brooks (1975), Fuld and Fisher (1977), Tsushima and Towne (1977), Levin and Eisenberg (1979), Rutter, Chadwick, Shaffer, and Brown (1980), Chadwick, Rutter, Thompson, and Shaffer (1980), Black, Blumer, Wellner, Shepart, and Walker (1981), Brown, Chadwick, Shaffer, Rutter, and Traub (1981), and Chadwick, Rutter, Brown, Shaffer, and Traub (1981).

Since 1966, head injuries have been one of the major areas of interest of a group of investigators at the University of British Columbia. This group included neuropsychologists, neurosurgeons, neurologists, electroencephalographers, pediatricians and psychiatrists. Varying aspects of head injuries of children, as well as

Table 1.   Categories of data obtained about the head injured child

	Neurologist/ Neurosurgeon	Neuro- Psychologist	Psychiatrist
1. Epidemiology and Natural History	X	X	
2. Historical-Personal			
(a) Child	X	X	X
(b) Parents	X	X	X
3. Educational			
(a) Child	X	X	X
(b) Parents	X	X	X
(c) School Records		X	
(d) Management		X	
4. Health			
(a) Premorbid status	X	X	X
(b) Management during acute and post-acute phases	X		
(c) EEG	X		
(d) Radiographic	X		
(e) Physical status	X		X
(f) Mental status	X	X	X
(g) Emotional status		X	X
(h) Neuropsychological status		X	
(i) Brain-behavior relationships		X	

adults, have been examined. In a clinical context, involving a
number of multidisciplinary projects, many hundreds of head-
injured children have been examined. Based on these extensive
observations, this chapter will provide an overview of the
research findings and the method of clinical management of the
head-injured child. First, a model will be presented from the
perspective of neuropsychology, which covers the gamut of concepts
and data from epidemiology to litigation.

MODEL OF NATURAL HISTORY OF HEAD INJURIES

The model to be delineated includes the salient variables
pertaining to the natural history of head injuries. The variables
identified in this model should assist in more effective management during the course of recovery, and also enable more precise
predictions about the nature of the long-term sequelae. First,
the model focuses on antecedent factors such as constitutional
predisposition, premorbid personality, age, sex, and environmental
hazards. Second, the model includes the circumstances at the time
of head injury, such as nature and extent of injury, resilience of
the neural apparatus in childhood, and the nature of intervention
and management during the acute and post-acute phases with particular emphasis on the neuropsychological examination. Third, the
model addresses consequence factors, such as the short and long-
term effects of head injury, with particular emphasis on neuropsychology, the effect of brain damage on general adaptation and
maturation, the probability of the development of post-traumatic
epilepsy, the effects of brain damage on education and transaction
with family, and the role of compensation and litigation. The
model also encompasses a variety of clinical examinations, including neurological, electroencephalographic, radiographic and neuropsychological. Finally, the model attempts to address the differentiation of immediate, short-term and long-term effects, as well
as the nature and course of recovery.

What data are required to make the necessary judgments about
the course of recovery from, and the prognosis of, head injuries
in children? In this same clinical context, it also can be asked,
what are the primary roles of professionals, especially that of
the neurosurgeon and/or neurologist, the psychologist or neuropsychologist, and the psychiatrist? Table 1 presents four groupings of data that are needed to answer the first question, and
the professional disciplines responsible for acquiring the information constituting the data base.

It can be seen that the first component of the data base
deals with epidemiology and natural history. The following
morbidity and mortality data derived from studies of head injuries
in children should sensitize the reader to the importance of this

Table 2.   Comparison of slight and more severe head-injured children

Method

1. Groups:

    a. emergency preschool

    b. emergency school

    c. emergency school control

    d. hospital preschool

    e. hospital school

    f. hospital school control

2. Sample: N=588

3. Age range: 0.2 to 16.1 years

4. Demographic characteristics:

    a. census tract

    b. race

    c. parents marital status

    d. occupation (father)

    e. occupation (mother)

    f. education (father)

    g. education (mother)

5. Developmental history and predisposing factors:

    a. premature birth

    b. development

    c. motor activity

    d. predisposing factors

6. Educational history:

    a. educational placement

    b. educational achievement

7. Accident proneness:

    a. previous accidents

    b. previous head injuries

8. Sequelae one year afeter accident

problem to health management (Chowdhary, 1978; Rosman, 1978; Moyes, 1980; Jennett & MacMillan, 1981).

Accidents are the major cause of childhood mortality and morbidity over the age of one; accidents are the leading cause of mortality in children between the ages of one and 14, of which a major portion involve trauma to the head; head injuries are the most frequent of all neuropediatric disorders; head injuries account for fifteen percent of all deaths in the 15-24 age group.

The second component of the data base deals with the systematic accumulation, within a developmental frame of reference, of historical information from both the child and his or her parents. The third component of the data base involves detailing the educational history. While parents and the injured child are the primary informants, it is critical to have access to objective information as well, such as report cards, or even more preferably, a complete school record. These school records may contain, in addition to the child's grades, the results of psychological examinations, such as the scores on standardized tests of intelligence and achievement. This information is especially useful in planning the return to school of the head-injured child and in advising school authorities about special management that would be required.

The fourth component of the data base concerns health status. During the acute phase, it is the neurosurgeon who is exclusively involved in management. The neuropsychologist and psychiatrist generally are involved during the post-acute phase.

SLIGHT AND SEVERE HEAD INJURIES

Methodology. Our first study compared children with slight head injuries to children with severe head injuries (Klonoff, 1971). The methodology and findings are presented in Tables 2 and 3, respectively. Subsequently, our most ambitious research project was undertaken involving a five-year follow-up study of 231 head-injured children who ranged in age from 3 to less than 16. Despite attrition over the six examination periods, neuropsychological, neurological and EEG measurements were obtained on 970 head-injured children, and repeated neuropsychological measurements were collected on 1050 normal controls (Klonoff & Paris, 1974; Klonoff & Low, 1974; Klonoff, Low, & Clark, 1977).

Neuropsychological sequelae. The results of the neuropsychological examination are summarized in Figure 1. The following should be noted: 1) for the younger group (ages 3 to less than 9) the initial cohort of 131 was reduced after five years to 75 subjects, while for the older group (ages 9 to less than 16) the initial cohort of 100 was reduced to 39 subjects. This attrition occurred despite our constant attempts to track, contact and arrange for return and re-examination; 2) the neuropsychological battery consisted of 18 tests and 32 variables for the younger group and 23 tests and 48 variables for the older group; 3) there was a more or less parallel pattern of generalized impairment during hospitalization for both the younger and the older head-injured children. Most of the reconstitution occurred by 2 years after the injury, but there were also continued gains 3 years after the injury, as well as a few significant improvements up to five years after the injury; 4) whereas both the younger and the older head-injured children had identical percentages of impairment among the test variables during the initial examination (87%), it was found that the older head-injured children had a higher percentage of impaired variables (12% vs. 3%) than the younger group after five years.

Table 3.   Summary of effects of head-injury in children

Results

1. Boys are more vulnerable than girls to suffering a head injury in a 12 to 7 ratio.

2. Children between the ages of less than 1 are most susceptible to head injury.

3. Accident proneness is significantly higher in boys.

4. No specific relationship exists between medical history (developmental anomalies, hyperactivity, mental deficiency, brain damage, emotional disturbance) and predisposition to head injury.

5. There is a significant relationship between type of environment (congested residential areas, lower income housing, marital instability, lower occupational status of father) and rate of head injury.

6. The sequelae for the younger children include: irritability and personality changes. Headaches, dizzy spells, impaired memory and learning difficulties characterize the older children.

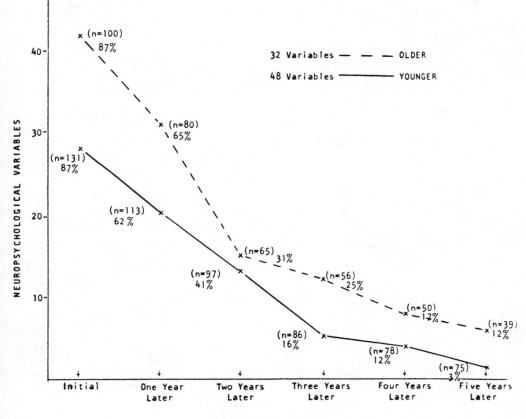

TIME   AFTER   INJURY

Fig. 1.   Comparison of young (<9) and older (9 –16) head–injured
children with matched controls on neuropsychological
variables – analysis of variance.

Table 4. Full-scale IQ on repeated examinations of head-injured and normal controls

	Initial	Follow-up				
		1st yr.	2nd yr.	3rd yr.	4th yr.	5th yr.
Head-injured	101.9	103.9	108.4	109.4	110.2	110.2
Normal-controls	113.9	114.9	116.8	118.4	118.8	118.3

Table 5. Full-scale IQ for each age level under nine on repeated examinations for head injured and normal controls

Age	n	Mean & S.D.	Initial	Follow-up				
				1st yr.	2nd yr.	3rd yr.	4th yr.	5th yr.
Head-injured								
3	13	$\bar{x}$	98.5	102.2	110.5	111.5	114.1	112.3
		s	13.8	13.8	10.0	10.0	9.4	7.7
4	12	$\bar{x}$	100.4	96.7	105.1	105.0	107.3	108.0
		s	18.4	12.7	12.9	14.5	14.5	14.8
5	17	$\bar{x}$	102.7	103.3	108.8	111.0	111.9	112.6
		s	16.7	14.2	12.1	13.4	12.3	14.9
6	10	$\bar{x}$	104.1	107.6	110.3	109.9	108.2	108.1
		s	17.6	14.7	14.1	14.9	13.9	13.2
7	10	$\bar{x}$	104.2	111.4	112.8	114.2	113.2	114.6
		s	6.2	8.9	10.4	9.7	7.0	11.0
8	14	$\bar{x}$	102.1	104.2	104.5	105.5	106.6	105.8
		s	10.9	10.2	10.5	10.6	9.4	8.6
Normal Controls								
3	11	$\bar{x}$	115.1	117.4	110.0	118.4	117.4	116.9
		s	8.9	8.6	6.9	8.3	9.9	8.7
4	18	$\bar{x}$	115.5	112.2	118.8	120.4	120.6	120.4
		s	10.9	10.9	9.8	11.3	10.5	9.7
5	18	$\bar{x}$	110.4	115.8	117.1	116.7	117.3	115.8
		s	10.0	10.6	11.2	10.6	8.7	9.8
6	13	$\bar{x}$	113.0	116.5	120.3	117.7	122.0	118.1
		s	8.3	7.2	8.1	8.8	10.7	9.6
7	9	$\bar{x}$	114.7	113.8	116.3	119.4	118.5	118.9
		s	7.2	5.5	5.9	9.8	6.5	5.4
8	14	$\bar{x}$	115.7	114.8	116.1	118.1	116.9	119.6
		s	7.5	5.8	6.4	8.1	9.6	10.4

An analysis of the intellectual changes in the children who were less than nine years of age reveals some interesting trends. Table 4 summarizes the five-year changes in IQ after trauma for the head-injured children and the control children using either the Stanford-Binet Intelligence Scale (children less than five years of age), or the Wechsler Intelligence Scale for Children (children between 5 and 9 years of age). Upon initial examination, it was observed that the children who had been head-injured were functioning in the average range; while the matched controls were functioning in the bright-normal range. Because of practice and maturation, the matched controls showed a 4.4 point increment in IQ after 5 years. Most of these gains were made during the first three annual re-examinations, with little change being noted during the next two re-examinations. In part, this reflects not only the ceiling effect of the test battery, but also indicates the limits of the effects of practice trials which are spaced one year apart. The head-injured children showed substantially the same trend, but with smaller gains being made during the first three years.

Table 5 summaries the intellectual changes for each age level between 3 and 8 for the six examinations. Upon comparing the head-injured and normal controls, the following trends are noted: 1) intellectual functioning at each examination point is the result of the effects of both reconstitution and practice; 2) the rate of change for the head-injured group is almost twice that of the normal controls - this improvement probably being due to the effects of reconstitution; 3) there is much more variability in the rate of change of intellectual functioning in the head-injured children, while others show only a 3-4 point change; and, 4) that the rate of change is almost evenly distributed among older and younger head-injured children.

In summary, the results of the analysis of the relationship between age level and intellectual functioning after head-injury indicate that the IQ is significantly lower compared to normal controls throughout the five-year examination period, and that this difference is most apparent during the initial and first-year follow-up. This may imply that intelligence scores obtained after head-injury cannot be used as a matching variable without incurring the risk of confounding seriously the results obtained. More importantly, the rapid recovery in intellectual functioning does not parallel the course of change reflected on neuropsychological test batteries, indicating that intelligence tests tap a different category of functioning. Finally, these results illustrate that longitudinal studies must take into account the effects of practice and learning over the course of repeated examinations.

Table 6. Distribution of the summed deviation scores*

Distribution	Older (n=39)		Younger (n=75)		Total (n=114)	
	Normal	Head-Injured	Normal	Head-Injured	Normal	Head-Injured
Worse performance (< -5)	1	8	4	19	5	27
Cutoff (-5 to 5)	34	31	70	55	104	86
Best performance (> 5)	4	0	1	1	1	1
Range	-7 to 8	-14 to 5	-9 to 6	-14 to 7	-9 to 8	-14 to 7

*From Klonoff et al., 1977. Head injuries in children: A prospective five year follow-up. Neurology, Neurosurgery, and Psychiatry 40:1211-1219. Reproduced with permission of the publisher.

Table 7. Full scale IQ means derived from cut-off points on 11 neuropsychological variables five years after head injury[1]*

Examination Points	Normal (n=114)	Head-Injured no residual (n=87)	Head-Injured residual (n=27)
Initial	114.8	105.7	92.3
After five years	120.4	116.4	98.9

[1]F-values for the ANOVA were: between groups F=97.9, p<0.001; between examinations F=41.8, p<0.001; group by examination F=3.05, p<0.05.

*From Klonoff et al., 1977. Head injuries in children: A prospective five year follow-up. Neurology, Neurosurgery, and Psychiatry 40:1211-1219. Reproduced with permission of the publisher.

Further analyses were conducted to determine if there existed a sub-group within the head-injured children who were significantly different from both the normal controls and from the majority of the head-injured children. For both the younger and older groups, the within-group variances for each variable (IQ excluded) were compared in order to determine if there were differences in the distribution of specific variables between the normal children and the head-injured groups on the last re-examination. The following variables from the Reitan Battery were identified in which the variance in the head-injured groups was three times greater than the variance in the normal groups. For the younger group these included: 1) Category; 2) Tapping non-dominant; 3) Speech Perception; 4) Trail Making total; 5) Tactual Performance Test total time; and, 5) Tactual Performance Test memory. In the older group the variables were: 1) Category; 2) Tapping non-dominant; 3) Speech Perception; 4) Trail Making total; 5) Tactual Performance Test total time; 6) Tactual Performance test memory; 7) Lateral Dominance; 8) Grooved Pegboard dominant; 9) Grooved Pegboard non-dominant; 10) Foot-Tapping dominant; and, 11) Foot-Tapping non-dominant.

Each head-injured and normal child was assigned a score on these 11 variables that was based on the means and standard deviations of the scores of a normal sample of 158 children. The scores were assigned according to whether the obtained value fell within one standard deviation above or below the mean, between 1 and 2 standard deviations above or below the mean, or fell beyond two standard deviations above or below the mean. If the head-injured and normal groups were equivalent, then the distribution of scores for each group should be more or less the same; that is, having a mean at or near zero. The results, presented in Table 6, clearly indicate that there was a subgroup of head-injured children who were different from both the normal children and from the majority of the head-injured children. In fact, 23.7% of the head-injured children performed so poorly that their score on this revised scale fell outside the cut-off point, while only 4.4% of the normal children obtained scores beyond the cut-off point.

The relationship between the summed deviation score based on the neuropsychological tests and the score on the intelligence test provides cross validation regarding the existence of subgroups within the head-injured sample. The mean intelligence scores for the normal children (n=114), head-injured children with no discernible evidence of residual neuropsychological effects (n=87), and head-injured children with evidence of residual neuropsychological effects (n=27), were compared during initial hospitalization and again five years later, using between and within group analysis of variance. Table 7 summarizes the results using Tukey's multiple comparisons: 1) all three groups were significantly different during the hospital admission interval; 2) the

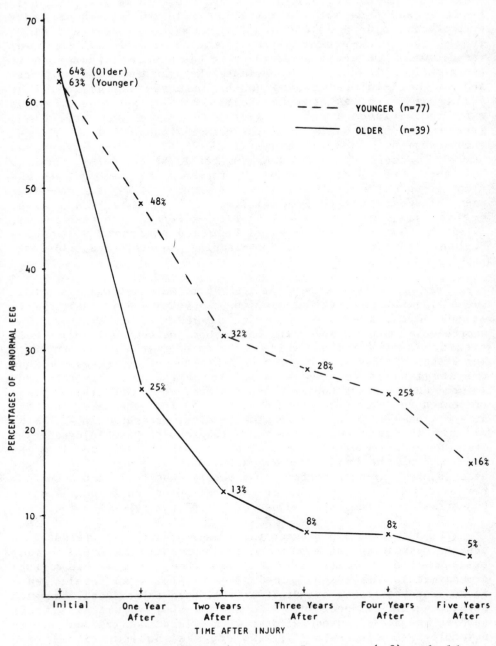

Fig. 2 EEG abnormal (Global) ratings for young (< 9) and older
(9 – 16) cohorts – in percentages.

head-injured group with no evidence of residual effects had a
significant increase in level of intellectual functioning from
hospital admission to the fifth follow-up examination, and five
years later, this group was no longer different from the normal
controls; 3) this latter group and the group of normal children
were both significantly different from the head-injured group with
evidence of residual neuropsychological effects at the fifth
follow-up. These findings indicate that level of intellectual
functioning following head injury should be regarded as a dependent variable rather than as a matching or control variable in the
assessment of head injury.

   EEG sequelae. The results of the EEG examination are summarized in Figure 2. The following should be noted: 1) as with the
neuropsychological findings, there is an identical incidence of
EEG abnormality during the post-acute phase for both the younger
and the older head-injured children; 2) in contrast to the neuropsychological findings, however, the course of EEG recovery is not
parallel for the younger and the older head-injured groups; 3) for
the older group, most of the reconstitution takes place by two
years after the injury; a comparable rate of reconstitution does
not occur until five years after injury for the younger age group;
and, 4) in contrast to the neuropsychological findings, five years
after injury, the younger head-injured children had a higher
incidence of residual EEG abnormalities.

   Neurological sequelae. The neurological sequelae are summarized in Table 8. It can be seen that there is an identical
incidence of neurological sequelae for both the younger and the
older head-injured children one year after injury, a finding that
is similar to the neuropsychological results. The course of reconstitution is more or less parallel for both groups, but five
years after injury, the younger head-injured children exhibited a
slightly higher incidence of sequelae (38% vs. 31%) than the older
children.

   An examination of self-reported neurological complaints for
the younger and the older head-injured children indicated that
they were not significantly different from each other at the one-
year follow-up. However, unlike the younger group, the older
group decreased their complaints after five years (x^2 = 4.18,
p<0.05). The drop in the incidence of self-reported neurological
complaints is best illustrated by the specific complaint of headaches. Between the first- and the fifth-year follow-up, the incidence of headaches decreased slightly for the younger group (24%
to 19%), and substantially, but not significantly (x^2 = 2.97,
p<.10) for the older group (28% to 10%). A similar trend was
found for a number of other areas, such as personality, learning,
mood and voluntary muscle control.

Table 8.   Neurological sequelae for children less than 9 and more than 9 years of age at admission and five years later*

Nature of Sequelae	After one year		After five years	
	<9 yr (n=78)	>9 yr (n=39)	<9 yr (n=78)	>9 yr (n=39)
Incidence of Sequelae (f+%)	35(45%)	18(46%)	30(38%)	12(31%)
Areas (f)[1]				
Neurological	12	3	7	3
Subjective	19	12	19	5
Personality	20	10	15	5
Intellectual	8	5	6	6

[1](f + %) = frequency and percentage of cohort showing positive signs

*From Klonoff et al., 1977.   Head injuries in children: A prospective five year follow-up. Neurology, Neurosurgery, and Psychiatry 40:1211-1219. Reproduced with permission of the publisher.

Prediction of sequelae.   The capacity to predict the long-term neurological sequelae of traumatic brain damage would be very helpful in better understanding how to clinically manage the head-injured child, as well as contribute to our knowledge of the effects of head injury.   To this end, an attempt was made to establish a *post hoc* model using stepwise multiple regression analysis to predict the residual sequelae found during the fourth and fifth follow-up.   The following predictor variables obtained during initial hospitalization were utilized: 1) age; 2) gestation period (premature birth); 3) retrograde amnesia; 4) post-traumatic amnesia; 5) period of unconsciousness; 6) neurological rating; 7) EEG rating; and, 8) Full Scale IQ.   The use of all these variables resulted in a significant multiple regression coefficient of 0.473 ($F = 3.96$, df = 8/108, $p<0.01$).   The rank order of variables contributing to the prediction of sequelae was as follows: Initial Full Scale I.Q., period of unconsciousness, post-traumatic amnesia, EEG rating, neurological rating, gestation period, retrograde amnesia, and age. The best predictive variable was the Full Scale IQ that was obtained during initial hospital admission ($F = 10.89$, df = 1/108, $p<0.01$), followed by the period of unconsciousness ($F = 2.98$, df = 1/108, $p<0.10$).

The ability to predict longer term neuropsychological sequelae would add still another dimension to the management of the head-injured child.   Using the variables described above, the performance of the two subgroups of head-injured children (the 27 children with positive signs of neuropsychological impairment and the 87 children with no positive signs) was examined using a step-wise discriminant analysis. These variables were able to correctly classify 84% of the subjects in the two groups. Initial Full Scale IQ, period of unconsciousness, and post-traumatic amnesia were the most highly relevant variables for predicting the neuropsychological deficits five years after head injury.

The prediction of long-term EEG sequelae was also undertaken using the eight variables obtained during initial hospitalization. All of the EEG tracings were assigned a global rating of either normal, borderline, minimally abnormal, moderately abnormal or markedly abnormal. The criteria for these ratings have been described by Klonoff and Low (1974). The EEG tracings were further classified as either unequivocally normal, equivocal, or abnormal. This rating schema provided another stable measure of EEG recovery. During the initial hospital admission, the incidence of EEG abnormality was identical for the younger (64.5%) and older (65.8%) groups. Both the number of younger ($x^2 = 35.2$, p<0.001) and the older subjects ($x^2 = 25.0$, p<0.001) who showed an abnormal EEG declined in the interim from the initial examination to the fifth-year follow-up. A discriminant analysis was computed using the eight initial trauma variables with group membership defined as the presence or absence of an abnormal EEG. The overall correct classification was 79.3%, indicating that these variables were predictive of the presence of residual deficits five years after injury.

Interaction of sequelae. Table 9 summarizes the incidence of head-injury effects five years after the accident. Twenty-three percent of the head-injured sample exhibited positive signs of impairment on the neuropsychological measures, compared to 12% having an abnormal EEG, and 24% having neurological signs of impairment. Of the children who exhibited positive neuropsychological signs, 48% also exhibited positive signs on either the EEG or on the neurological examination. By way of contrast, of those with abnormal EEGs, 64% exhibited positive signs on examination using neuropsychological or neurological techniques. Among the children who demonstrated positive neuro-logical sequelae, only 43% had residual signs on the other examinations. Thus, there is a moderate degree of concordance between the neuropsychological, neurological and EEG realms of data.

These clinical findings of the residual effects of head-injury can be cross-validated with school performance. Hence, of the 33 children in both groups who were failing in school, or were in remedial class placement, 67% had documented effects in at least one area at the fifth follow-up.

The degree of concordance between the neuropsychological, EEG and neurological variables in this study does not differ from that found in investigations of adult head injuries. For example, the study by Tsushima and Wedding (1979) of adult head-injured patients showed a high degree of concordance between the neurological diagnosis and the percentage of head trauma patients correctly diagnosed with CT Scan, EEG, and two measures of the Halstead-Reitan Battery. Yet, it should be realized that each procedure has its own base rate of abnormality and rates of accuracy. Physical examination (Stuss & Trites, 1977), and X-ray (Filskov & Goldstein, 1974) appear to have rather low rates of accuracy for identification and lateralization of neuropathological processes, while the brain scans (Christie, Mori, Go, Cornell, & Schapiro, 1976) and blood flow measures (Lassen, Ingevar, & Skinhoj, 1978) appear to be more accurate. However, it should be noted that the parameters measured by these different procedures are somewhat independent, and thus, brain-damaged patients need not necessarily show abnormalities on all of these procedures.

Table 9. Overall assessment of head injury effects*

Area/Subject	Positive Signs of Impairment	
	Number	Percent
By Area		
Neuropsychological	27	23.0
EEG	14	12.0
Neurological	28	23.9
By Subject		
Number exhibiting	51	43.6
One area only	35	29.9
Two areas	14	12.0
Three areas	2	1.7

*From Klonoff et al., 1977. Head injuries in children: A prospective five year follow-up. Neurology, Neurosurgery, and Psychiatry 40:1211-1219. Reproduced by permission of the publisher.

THE NEUROPSYCHOLOGIST AS AN EXPERT WITNESS

McMahon and Satz (1981) have provided a systematic review of the application of neuropsychology in a forensic context-criminal, as well as civil. Our intention is to focus on the area of personal injury litigation, and more specifically, on accidents which have involved head injury.

The neuropsychologist must recognize and accept the adversarial basis of the judicial system with the defined legal prerogatives of the plaintiff and the defendant. The neuropsychologist, regardless of whether the request for examination emanates from the attorney of the plaintiff or the defendant, must function within the prescribed code of ethics of the American Psychological Association. Furthermore, the neuropsychologist must recognize that in the arena of litigation he must abide by rules of procedure without compromising his professional and personal integrity. Giving evidence and in particular maintaining professional decorum during cross-examinations are learned roles, and the neuropsychologist is accordingly well advised to obtain the requisite training for an expert witness.

Credibility as an expert witness, however, derives from the scope of the examination and established expertise as a neuropsychologist, and not from posturing in a courtroom. Hence, the model of the natural history of head injuries covered in this presentation is a prerequisite for conceptualizing the ramifications of a head injury.

The neuropsychologist's data base should include the following:

1. **Intellectual-Neuropsychological Status**
    a. current level, pre-morbid level, prognosis;
    b. outstanding areas of cognitive and psychological deficits;
    c. relationship between practice effect and reconstitution;
    d. prognosis in terms of education; and,
    e. prognosis in terms of vocation/career.

2. **Emotional Status**
    a. current status, pre-morbid personality, prognosis;
    b. the presence and role of anxiety, depression, denial;
    c. coping mechanisms regarding physical-psychological trauma and educational-interpersonal demands; and,
    d. specific trauma deriving from death of family member.

3. **Degree of Impairment**
    a. extensity scale in terms of minimal-moderate-extensive;
    b. impairment includes intellectual, personality, and physical parameters;

    c.   post-traumatic epilepsy occurs in 5% of closed head in-
         juries and the incidence is much higher in open-head in-
         juries. This is an important factor in determining
         impairment;

    d.   the presence of unremitting aphasia is another important
         factor in determining degree of impairment;

    e.   head injuries are not infrequently in a context of
         multiple injuries (e.g., hemiparesis or quadraplegia) and
         form a very important consideration in determining impair-
         ment in a global sense.

REFERENCES

Black, P., Blumer, D., Wellner, A.M. & Walker, A.E. The head-
injured child: Time-course of recovery, with implications for
rehabilitation. Sec. V. In: **Head injuries, proceedings of an
international symposium.** Edinburgh and London, Churchill
Livingstone, 1971.

Black, P., Blumer, D., Wellner, A.M., Shepart, R.H., & Walker,
A.E. Head trauma in children: Neurological, behavioral, and
intellectual sequelae. In: P. Black (Ed.), **Brain dysfunction
in children: Etiology, diagnosis and management.** New York:
Raven, 1981.

Brink, J.D., Garrett, A.L., Hale, W.R., Woo-Sam, J., & Nickel,
V.L. Recovery of motor and intellectual function in children
sustaining severe head injuries. **Developmental Medicine &
Child Neurology**, 1970, 12, 565-571.

Brown, F., Chadwick, O., Shaffer, D., Rutter, M., & Traub, M. A
prospective study of children with head injuries: III. Psychiatric sequelae. **Psychological Medicine**, 1981, 11, 63-78.

Chadwick, O., Rutter, M., Thompson, J., & Shaffer, D. Intellectual performance and reading skills after localized head injury
in childhood. **Journal of Child Psychology & Psychiatry**, 1980,
22, 117-139.

Chadwick, O., Rutter, M., Brown, G., Shaffer, D. & Traub, M. A
prospective study of children with head injuries: II. Cognitive sequelae. **Psychological Medicine**, 1981, 11, 49-61.

Christie, J., Mori, H., Go, R., Cornell, S., & Schapiro, R. Computed tomography and radionuclide studies in the diagnosis of
intercranial diseases. **American Journal of Reontgenology**,
1976, **127**, 171-174.

Chowdhary, U.M. Comparative epidemiology of head injuries in developed and developing countries. **Journal Irish Medical Association**, 1978, 71, 617-620.

Filskov, S. & Goldstein, S. Diagnostic validity of the Halstead-
Reitan Neuropsychological Battery. **Journal of Consulting &
Clinical Psychology**, 1974, 42, 382-388.

Fuld, P.A. & Fisher, P. Recovery of intellectual ability after
closed head injury. **Developmental Medicine & Child Neurology**,
1977, 19, 495-502.

Jennett, B. & MacMillan, R. Epidemiology of head injury. **British Medical Journal**, 1981, **282**, 101–104.

Klonoff, H. Head injuries in children: Predisposing factors, accident conditions, accident proneness and sequelae. **American Journal of Public Health**, 1971, **61**, 198–213.

Klonoff, H. & Low, M. Disordered brain function in young children and early adolescents: Neuropsychological and electroencephalographic correlates. In R. Reitan & L.A. Davison, (Eds.), **Clinical neuropsychology: Current status and applications.** New York: John Wiley & Sons, 1974.

Klonoff, H., Low, M.D., & Clark, C. Head injuries in children: A prospective five-year follow-up. **Journal of Neurology, Neurosurgery & Psychiatry**, 1977, **40**, 1211–1219.

Klonoff, H. & Paris, R. Immediate, short-term and residual effects of acute head injuries in children: Neuropsychological and neurological correlates. In R. Reitan & L.A. Davison (Eds.), **Clinical neuropsychology: Current status and applications.** New York: John Wiley & Sons, 1974.

Lassen, N., Ingevar, D., & Skinhoj, E. Brain function and blood flow. **Scientific American**, 1978, **239**, 62–71.

Levin, H. & Eisenberg, H. Neuropsychological outcome of closed head injury in children and adolescents. **Child's Brain**, 1979, **5**, 281–292.

Mandelberg, I.A. & Brooks, D.N. Cognitive recovery after head injury. **Journal of Neurology, Neurosurgery & Psychiatry**, 1975, **38**, 1121–1126.

Moyes, C.D. Epidemiology of serious head injuries in childhood. **Child: Care, Health & Development**, 1980, **6**, 1–9.

Rutter, M., Chadwick, O., Shaffer, D., & Brown, G. A prospective study of children with head injuries: 1. design and methods. **Psychological Medicine**, 1980, **10**, 633–645.

Rosman, N.P. Pediatric head injuries. **Pediatric Annals**, 1978, **7**, 55–74.

Stuss, E. & Trites, R. Classification of neurological status using multiple discriminant function analysis of neuropsychological test scores. **Journal of Consulting & Clinical Psychology**, 1977, **45**, 145.

Tsushima, W. & Towne, W.S. Neuropsychological abilities of young children with questionable brain disorders. **Journal of Consulting & Clinical Psychology**, 1977, **45**, 757–762.

Tsushima, W.T. & Wedding, D. A comparison of the Halstead-Reitan neuropsychological battery and computerized tomography in the identification of brain disorder. **Journal of Nervous and Mental Disease**, 1979, **167**, 704–707.

NEUROPSYCHOLOGICAL ASPECTS OF CHILDHOOD EPILEPSY

Lawrence Hartlage

Medical College of Georgia
Department of Neurology
Augusta, Georgia

and

Cathy Fultz Telzrow

Cuyahoga Special Education Service Center
Cleveland, Ohio

The period of modern research in epilepsy often is dated to J. Hughlings Jackson's conceptualization of the epileptic seizure as a sudden and violent discharge of brain cells (Dreifus, 1975), an explanation which is essentially the same as that used today. With the introduction and common use of the electroencephalograph (EEG) in 1929 (Millikan, 1976), the ability to study seizure activity more directly was greatly advanced. As a result of the development and use of anticonvulsant medications since World War II ("Epilepsy," 1980), as well as comprehensive investigations into the psychosocial (Bagley, 1971; Dodrill et al., 1980) and vocational (Hedgeman, 1978) aspects of individuals with epilepsy, our understanding of this condition has increased significantly.

Current estimates place the incidence of epilepsy anywhere from one to four percent of the population (Wright, 1975). Of the two million Americans with epilepsy, the greatest proportion are children (Millikan, 1976). It has been estimated that as many as 4% of all children experience at least one seizure prior to the age of fifteen (Dodson et al., 1976a). Seventy-five percent of all cases of epilepsy begin before age 18 ("Plan for Nationwide Action," 1977). While the number of children with epilepsy marks it as a major medical problem, factors such as the effects of cumulative seizures on cognitive and emotional development, the consequences of long-term use of anti-convulsant medications, and the disrupted psychosocial environment of the child with seizures all underscore the seriousness of this condition.

In order to make a discussion of neuropsychological aspects of childhood epilepsy meaningful, the initial sections of this chapter will focus on definition, classification, diagnosis, and prevalence of childhood epilepsy. Next, the chapter will address the mental development and behavioral characteristics of children with epilepsy. A discussion of the various therapies and interventions that are in common use will conclude the chapter.

DEFINITION

The term "epilepsy" is applied to the condition in which repeated seizures occur without apparent cause. Because certain conditions, such as alcohol and drug excess, as well as sleep deprivation, can precipitate seizures in otherwise non-epileptic individuals, this distinction is critical. Although clinicians tend to vary in their inclination to diagnose epilepsy where there are only isolated seizure episodes (Robb, 1972; Millikan, 1976), the diagnosis is generally made only after a history of seizures is substantiated (Rodin, 1975).

Rodin (1975) notes that epileptic seizures are both involuntary and short lived. With the exception of status epilepticus, which is the term given to prolonged, unbroken episodes of multiple convulsions, seizures usually do not extend beyond 90 seconds (Millikan, 1976). Seizures accompanied by a loss or alteration in consciousness are generally similar in a given individual, and are characterized by meaningless, repetitive behaviors or movements (Rodin, 1975). It is clear that epilepsy is not a disease, but rather reflects an underlying condition of which the seizures represent one symptom. The underlying cause(s) and the manifestation of the seizures are themselves highly varied, thereby making epilepsy a complex condition and not a unitary syndrome ("Plan for Nationwide Action," 1977).

DIAGNOSIS

It should be evident from the above discussion that the diagnosis of epilepsy may not be a simple or straightforward matter. Many epileptic seizures are not of the tonic-clonic or *grand mal* type, although these represent the stereotyped seizure in the layman's imagination. Unlike many other disorders, epilepsy is unusual in that most of the time the symptom is not present (Townsend, 1976). Unless the person is hospitalized so that continual EEG monitoring is possible, rarely will the physician actually witness a seizure. Thus, a diagnosis must be made without the direct ob-

servation of the primary symptomatology. Most clinicians agree
that the patient's history is the single most valuable diagnostic
variable (Penry & Newmark, 1979).

Although the EEG has contributed significantly to the diagnosis of epilepsy, nearly 20% of persons with recurrent seizures
do not have abnormal EEG readings (Harris, 1976). Conversely, it
has been estimated that 25% of persons who are otherwise without
symptoms have abnormal EEG tracings (Kaufman, 1981). Furthermore,
numerous neuropathological conditions may result in similarly
distorted EEGs (Millikan, 1976). Nevertheless, the EEG is an
important diagnostic tool, especially for the identification of
childhood epilepsy, since a complete history may be more difficult
to obtain in this population (Millikan, 1976).

Another diagnostic issue concerns the phenomenon of hyster-
ical or pseudo-seizures. A recent study of 60 selected patients
with seizures revealed that 12 (20%) experienced *only* pseudo-
seizures during the in-hospital test condition. The majority of
these (83%) were receiving treatment with anti-convulsant medications on the basis of their pseudo-seizures (King et al., 1982).
These findings support the results obtained by Jeavons (1975), who
reported that 20% of 420 patients seen at two epileptic clinics
were not epileptic.

PREVALENCE

The lack of clarity in both the definition and diagnosis of
epilepsy makes any statement about the prevalence rate equivocal
at best (Robb, 1972). The rates reported range from .35% (Hauser
& Kurland, 1972) to 6.6% (Metrakos & Metrakos, 1960), depending
upon the nature of the populations, the diagnostic criteria, and
other factors. Prevalence rates are typically higher in child
than in adult populations (Millikan, 1976). In a study of nearly
12,000 children between the ages of 5 and 14, Rutter and his
colleagues (1970) reported a prevalence rate of .7% for epilepsy.
The most commonly used figure, approximately two million Americans, represents 1% of the population (Millikan, 1976), and while
it has been shown to be found slightly more often in males (Rutter
et al., 1970; Hauser & Kurland, 1972; Robb, 1972), it is generally
thought to be distributed approximately equally across the sexes
(Millikan, 1976).

CLASSIFICATION

In 1970, an international classification system of epileptic
seizures was adopted by the International League Against Epilepsy
("Plan for Nationwide Action," 1977). This classification schema,
based on descriptions of seizure type, has been widely accepted by

the scientific communities in most countries, and is generally employed in the epilepsy literature (see Table 1).

The two major categories of seizure types are: 1) generalized seizures, which affect the brain as a whole; and, 2) partial seizures, which involve only a discrete portion of the brain. Generalized seizures are of two major types. Absences, previously known as *petit mal* seizures, are characterized by a few seconds of

Table 1.   International Classification System of Epileptic Seizures

I.   Partial Seizures (beginning locally)
    A.   With elementary symptomatology; generally no impairment of consciousness
       1.   With motor symptoms (focal motor, Jacksonian, postural, involving speech, etc.)
       2.   With special sensory or somatosensory symptoms (visual, auditory, olfactory, gustatory, etc.)
       3.   With autonomic symptoms
       4.   Compound forms
    B.   With complex symptomatology; generally accompanied by impairment of consciousness
       1.   With impairment of consciousness only
       2.   With cognitive/intellectual symptomatology
       3.   With affective symptomatology
       4.   With psychomotor symptomatology (automatisms)
       5.   With psychosensory symptomatology (illusions/hallucinations)
       6.   Compound forms
    C.   Secondarily generalized partial seizures

II. Generalized Seizures
    A.   Absences (petit mal)
       1.   Impairment of consciousness only
       2.   Impairment of consciousness and associated phenomena (clonic components, automatisms, etc.)
    B.   Myoclonic jerks
    C.   Infantile spasms
    D.   Clonic seizures
    E.   Tonic-seizures
    F.   Tonic-clonic seizures
    G.   Atonic seizures
    H.   Akinetic seizures

III. Unilateral Seizures

IV. Unclassified Seizures

staring, lip smacking and eye blinking, but not a loss of consciousness. Absences occur primarily in children below age fifteen (Kaufman, 1981), and often occur several times daily. In spite of their typical frequency, absences are often unnoticed by parents and teachers because of their quiet, undramatic character- istics (Ansbaugh et al., 1980). The diagnosis of absences gener- ally can be confirmed by an EEG examination, since affected in- dividuals characteristically reveal a three-cycle-per second fre- quency pattern on the EEG (Kaufman, 1981).

The second type of generalized seizure, the tonic-clonic type (previously known as *grand mal* seizures), is the dramatic, stereo- typed seizure that is usually portrayed in the popular litera- ture. The tonic component of the seizure occurs when violent neuronal discharges produce extreme contraction of muscles, loss of consciousness, rapid expiration of breath that results in the "epileptic cry," blue skin color, and accumulation of saliva in and around the mouth. The clonic phase follows, and is character- ized by rhythmic spasmodic jerking of the previously rigid muscles toward the midline. Although the entire tonic-clonic seizure generally lasts only several seconds, there may be impaired con- sciousness, agitation, and deep sleep for up to several hours afterward. Sometimes a temporary hemiparesis may occur following the seizure (Millikan, 1976). The dramatic nature of the tonic- clonic seizure makes the history of superstition surrounding epi- lepsy comprehensible. Absences and tonic-clonic seizures are not mutually exclusive, and it has been reported that persons with absence seizures generally experience at least one tonic-clonic episode per year (Kaufman, 1981).

Unlike generalized seizures, partial seizures appear to be circumscribed to a focal area of the brain. Partial seizures may have motor or sensory symptoms, dependent upon the locus of the underlying abnormal brain tissue. The patient does not lose con- sciousness during partial seizures, although consciousness may be altered, and a dream-like or trance-like demeanor may be present. Partial seizures may have simple or complex symptomatology, and seizure behavior may vary from a simple peripheral motor movement (e.g., finger or foot twitching) to visual, auditory, or olfactory hallucinations (Dreifuss, 1975).

Nearly half of all children with seizures have been reported to demonstrate only tonic-clonic seizures; while three percent have exclusively absence seizures (Rutter et al., 1970). Most children experience a variety of seizure types during a given period (Millikan, 1976). In addition, certain seizure types are clearly age-related, so that a given child may demonstrate a vari- ation in seizures during his or her lifetime (Dreifuss, 1975). Often children who have absences while young will become seizure- free after about age fifteen, although approximately one-half of

the children with absences subsequently develop tonic-clonic seizures (Kaufman, 1981).

ETIOLOGY

When examining the causes of epilepsy, one must distinguish
the immediate or proximal cause from the distal, or etiological
condition. The proximal cause of epilepsy is abnormal electrical
discharges in the brain. Thus, it can be stated conclusively that
the immediate or proximal cause of epilepsy is abnormal brain
functioning. Of more significance, however, are the etiological
factors associated with this abnormal electrical discharge.

Harris (1976) described three conditions that are relevant to
the manifestation of epilepsy. The first condition, a constitutional predisposition to seizures, may be genetically determined.
Evidence for the heritability of vulnerability for epilepsy has
been reported (Andermann, 1979; Droose, 1979), including those
epilepsies that are due to biochemical disorders and enzyme
defects (Dreifuss, 1975). Metrakos and Metrakos (1960) found that
the siblings of children with generalized seizures had a 10%
chance of developing epilepsy, a risk level that is substantially
higher than the general population.

The second factor cited by Harris (1976) which relates to the
development of epilepsy is an epileptogenic focus in the brain.
This focus may occur as a result of trauma; perinatal hypoxia that
results in seizure types commonly known as temporal lobe epilepsy
or mesial temporal sclerosis (Harris, 1976; Polkey, 1976; Taylor,
1976); improper development of the brain due to toxic substances
or infections (Dreifuss, 1975); or a neoplasm or intracranial
tumor (Taylor, 1976). The third and final factor Harris (1976)
associated with the onset of seizure disorders is a precipitating
event or condition. This may take several forms, including stimulation by certain visual patterns or internal states such as
sleeplessness or hunger. Stress also has been linked to the onset
of seizures in susceptible individuals (Millikan, 1976). In addition, activation of seizures for the purpose of diagnosis often
can be induced by hyperventilation and photic stimulation
(Millikan, 1976). A fascinating series of studies on the various
types of reflex epilepsies has been reported by Forster (1977),
who has documented how certain seizures are provoked by eating,
reading unfamiliar material aloud, making decisions as in a chess
game, and writing without visual input.

Although numerous etiological factors have been identified
(e.g., head trauma, biochemical disorders, perinatal hypoxia, certain disease syndromes such as tuberous sclerosis), it is important to note that for the largest number of cases, no etiology can
be implicated (Ajmone-Marson, & Ralston, 1957; "Epilepsy," 1980).

Often in cases where there is no detectable physiological or anatomical abnormality (idiopathic epilepsy), there is a family history of the syndrome (Lezak, 1976).

MENTAL DEVELOPMENTAL CHARACTERISTICS

Several factors contaminate research on the mental development characteristics of children with epilepsy. As has been
emphasized previously, epilepsy is not a unitary condition with
singular expression, etiology and severity, but rather a culmination from a complex interactive network of these various dimensions. Thus, an epileptic population represents a heterogeneous
group for whom generalizations are at best difficult. Questions
related to the primary type of seizure experienced, age of seizure
onset, frequency of seizure episodes, and occurrence of status
epilepticus are significant when interpreting the literature
related to the mental development characteristics of epileptic
children. The research is complicated further by the potential
effects of numerous anti-convulsant medications, upon which a
large number of children with seizures rely for seizure control.

While recognizing these limitations, several statements
regarding the intellectual and academic performance of children
with epilepsy can be made. Studies generally have shown that
nearly half of epileptics have some degree of intellectual disability or impairment ("Plan for Nationwide Action," 1977). Rodin
et al. (1976) reported that 75% of persons with seizure disorders
demonstrate at least some impairment in intellectual, academic, or
behavioral performance.

Investigations into the distribution of intelligence in the
population of persons with epilepsy have revealed mixed results.
Several studies of intellectual ability reported that there is a
different distribution of intelligence scores for the epileptic
population than for non-epileptic controls. Rodin et al. (1976)
found that 30% of the epileptic population had IQs normal or
above, an additional 31% had IQs in the dull normal range, with
the remaining group (39%) falling in the borderline or defective
categories. These findings are generally supported by Bagley
(1971), who reported a mean IQ for epileptics comparable to that
of the general population, but a significantly skewed distribution, with substantially more of the epileptic subjects included
in the below-average portion of the distribution. Contradictory
findings were reported by Rutter et al. (1970), who found a distribution of intelligence in epileptic children which closely ap-
proximates the distribution in normals. It is important to note,
however, that nearly all the epileptic children in their study
attended normal schools, as opposed to special schools or special
education classes, suggesting that the children in their sample
may have been less debilitated than other epileptic children.

The ability of the school environment to predict the IQ level of epileptic children was demonstrated by Halstead (1957), who found that the intellectual level of children with epilepsy is associated with the type of educational environment (e.g., special school versus normal school). It seems likely that epileptic children with lower IQs may be placed disproportionately in special schools. In addition, it is conceivable that the effect of a homogeneous special school environment may depress the IQ of epileptic children (Carlberg & Kavale, 1980).

Numerous studies have reported that the mean IQ of epileptic children, disregarding distribution, is below average. A recent study of 61 children with major motor epilepsy revealed a mean IQ of 84 (Dean, in press). Halstead (1957) found that the mean IQ of children with epilepsy was significantly lower than controls, and that within the epileptic population, children attending residential facilities had a significantly lower IQ than children in normal classrooms. Dodrill (1981b) concluded that persons with idiopathic epilepsy have slightly, though consistently, higher IQs than those for whom the etiological factors have been determined. In the majority of studies reviewed for this chapter, summarized in Table 2, the reported mean IQ for epileptics was subnormal.

Dennerll et al. (1964) reported a mean WAIS or WISC IQ of 89 in a population of 100 epileptic children, with the Verbal IQ (91.8) being significantly higher than the performance IQ (87.7). Factor analysis of the WISC identified three factors that were labelled verbal comprehension, perceptual organization, and distractibility. It is interesting to note that these three factors also have been identified in normal children who were tested on the WISC-R (Kaufman, 1979). In addition, learning disabled children typically have been found to demonstrate their poorest performance on the WISC-R subtests (Digit Span, Arithmetic, and Coding) that load on distractibility (Kaufman, 1979). It seems feasible to infer that both epileptic and learning disabled children have deficits which implicate neurological impairment.

In addition to the studies of general intellectual capacity, research has focussed on the specific patterns of intellectual performance. Gastaut (1964) reported that over one-third of a group of epileptic children with IQs above 80 demonstrated perceptual-motor deficits. In comparing performance of brain-injured children with controls on a variety of tasks, Boll (1972) found that motor speed was one of the least impaired aspects of functioning. Cognitive functioning was most deficient in brain-injured children, followed by visual perception, auditory perception, motor speed and tactile form perception. Boll et al. (1978) subsequently demonstrated that brain-injured children who performed poorly on a perceptual tactile measure also had low achievement test scores. The authors suggest, as have others, that sensory and motor functions predict academic performance.

Another type of impairment observed in epileptic children appears to have its substrate in the left hemisphere, and is characterized by varying forms of language impairment. Cooper and Ferry (1978) reviewed cases of acquired aphasia associated with seizures in children. These seizures appear to occur more frequently in males, and even after they are controlled successfully, may be associated with substantial language disturbance. Adults who have partial seizures may demonstrate a transient aphasia or "speech arrest" which clears following the seizure episode (Gilmore & Heilman, 1981). Restitution to previous functioning does not, however, appear to occur in children, thus underscoring the vulnerability of the developing brain.

Fedio and Mirsky (1969) report that disorders of attention and constructional apraxia occur most frequently in children with generalized epilepsy. Children with temporal lobe epilepsy demonstrate patterns of impairment that are specific to the hemisphere involved: left temporal foci being associated with deficits in verbal learning, while right temporal abnormalities result in problems in the acquisition and recall of nonverbal material (Fedio & Mirsky, 1969). While the lesion site in epilepsy is correlated with degree and type of intellectual impairment (Vogel & Broverman, 1964), it is noteworthy that the EEG classification of a lesion focus does not accurately predict either intellectual capacity or academic performance (Hartlage & Green, 1973).

Considering the tendency toward depressed intellectual capacity, it is not surprising that the academic performance of epileptic children often is below average (Boll et al., 1978). Goldin et al. (1971) report especially poor academic performance by epileptic children who have additional disabilities. Numerous studies demonstrated that even after an adjustment for IQ is made, the achievement levels of epileptic children had lower than expected reading levels, with 18% of the subjects being at least two years below their expected level. Green and Hartlage (1971) found that the academic performance of epileptic children and adolescents was below anticipated levels. They suggested that this may have reflected in part the influence of lowered parental expectations. Reduced demands by teachers also may be a contributing factor to the underachievement of epileptic children (Ansbaugh et al., 1980).

The association of seizure frequency with degree of intellectual impairment also has been investigated (Dreifuss, 1975). In one study relating the number of seizures to intellectual and psychosocial development, Dodrill (1981a) divided subjects into four groups based on the total number of lifetime seizures and exis-

tence of status epilepticus. Group 1 comprised individuals who
had between 2 and 19 seizures; Group 2 included individuals who
had between 11-100 seizures; and, Group 3 persons reported more
than 100 seizures. None of the individuals in these groups had a
history of status epilepticus. Group 4 comprised individuals who
reported status epilepticus regardless of the number of seizure
episodes. The findings revealed that Groups 1 and 2 had the high-
est performance on the intellectual measures (WAIS). No significant differences were noted between these two groups, and both
performed better than Groups 3 and 4. Seidenberg et al. (1981)
used a test-retest paradigm to investigate intellectual functioning in a group of epileptic patients. At the time of retest, the
sample was divided into two groups according to whether or not
there was a decrease or increase in seizures. The interval between testings was approximately 18 months. For the unimproved
group, just one subtest (Block Design) and the Performance IQ on
the WAIS demonstrated a significant change in the positive direction. In contrast, the improved seizure group showed significant
gains on Full Scale, Performance and Verbal IQs, as well as on all
but three subtests (Arithmetic, Vocabulary and Digit Span). The
authors also found that while a decrease in seizure frequency was
associated with improvement in intellectual performance, an analysis of individual patient performance in the "no change" group
suggested intellectual deterioration.

Although both of the above studies tested adult subjects, and
caution must be exerted in extrapolating these findings to children, the implications for children are nonetheless provocative.
For example, postmortem investigations have revealed that ongoing
and uncontrolled seizure activity in adults is associated with
progressive loss of brain tissue (Dodson et al., 1976a). It is
reasonable that such pathology contributes to the deterioration of
intellectual functioning in children. A recent study of the effects of seizure frequency on neuropsychological performance of
children (Dean, in press) revealed significant negative correlations between the number of seizures and WISC scores. However, it
must be emphasized that deterioration is a complex process resulting from numerous factors, such as age of seizure onset (Dodrill,
1981b), premorbid intellectual performance, and nature and frequency of seizures (Dodrill, 1981a).

BEHAVIORAL CHARACTERISTICS

It is necessary to begin this section with the same dis-
claimer offered in the previous discussion; namely, epilepsy is a
heterogeneous and highly variable disorder with numerous manifestations and permutations. Unequivocal statements about the behavioral characteristics, therefore, are not possible, although
various trends can be described. Furthermore, anti-convulsant
medications affect the behavior of epileptic children such that it

is not readily possible to separate the influence of drugs from the epileptic mechanisms.

Personality changes in epileptics have long been hypothesized (Tizzard, 1962; Hermann, 1977). Lisansky (1948) reported that research which focussed on personality changes due to epilepsy implicated essentially three etiological factors: cerebral changes, environmental stresses, and a combination of these two variables. Evidence for cerebral alterations, which in turn result in personality changes, has been presented by numerous researchers, particularly for temporal lobe epilepsy, where personality changes appear most frequently (Geschwind et al., 1980). The second etiological mechanism postulated by Lisansky, environmental stress, has been studied extensively by Dodrill (1980, 1981b; Dodrill et al., 1980), who demonstrated major psychosocial deficits in epileptics. The interaction hypothesis, in which both environmental and organic factors contribute to the development of personality disturbances, also has been supported by research (Ritchie, 1981). Dodrill (1980), in examining the nature of this interaction, found that the severity of neuropsychological impairment was related to the degree of psychosocial maladjustment. Taylor (1976) found a similar relationship in temporal lobe epilepsy.

The relationship between epilepsy and psychopathology in children has received much attention. Nearly all of the studies cited have observed that the incidence of psychiatric disturbance in children with epilepsy exceeds the incidence in nonepileptic children. Pond and Bidwell (1960) reported that one-fourth of school-aged epileptic children demonstrated some degree of psychopathology. Rutter et al. (1970) found that psychopathology is 3 to 10 times more common in children with seizure disorders than in the general population, the exact prevalence depending on the particular type of seizure. The finding that the prevalence of psychiatric disturbance in epileptic children is at least twice that of children with physically handicapping conditions indicates that the psychopathology is related to the seizure and not general disability (Rutter et al., 1970).

A relationship between IQ and psychiatric disturbance also has been noted by Rutter et al. (1970). They observed that the prevalence of psychopathology was 50% in children who had intellectual impairment. In addition, a relationship has been observed between the severity of intellectual impairment and the type of behavioral disturbance. For example, Rutter et al. (1970) found a decidedly different pattern of psychiatric disturbance in brighter brain-damaged children who attended a regular school than a group of children who had been excluded from school because of severe intellectual impairment. The nature of the disturbance in the former group tended to take forms such as anxiety and aggression,

while the group of excluded children were more likely to demonstrate psychotic and hyperkinetic features.

One behavioral characteristic reported to occur widely in
epileptic children is hyperactivity (Ives, 1970). Ounsted (1955)
identified hyperactivity in 8% of a sample of epileptic children.
Hyperactivity also has been found to occur more frequently in
epileptic children with low IQs (Pond, 1961). There is also some
evidence that hyperactivity occurs with greater frequency in
younger epileptic children (Dreifuss, 1975). In addition, hyperactivity and an associated behavior, inattentiveness, are more
frequently found in boys with epilepsy, while the prevalence rates
for girls are comparable to nonepileptic children (Stores et al.,
1978).

There is some evidence linking the cerebral locus to the type
of manifest psychopathology. Watts (1975) noted that children
with bilateral amygdala lesions, such as those found in severe
cases of mesial temporal sclerosis, lack the ability to control
their emotions. Nuffield (1961) reported that temporal lobe epilepsy in children often is associated with aggressive behavior.
Bagley (1971), on the other hand, found that aggressive behavior
was more likely in persons who had nonspecific brain damage rather
than a temporal lobe focus. Recently, Hughes and Olsen (1981)
reported that there are distinguishable behavioral characteristics
that result from eight different temporal lobe loci. Geschwind et
al. (1980) have suggested that the temporal lobe epilepsies occasionally may be diagnosed on the basis of dramatic changes in behavior (such as preoccupation with sexuality, religiosity, and
hypergraphia). Further evidence linking temporal lobe foci with
behavioral disturbances can be found in studies reporting improved
behavioral functioning after temporal lobectomy (Williams, 1979).

Rutter et al. (1970) and Bagley (1971) reported that there is
no relationship between the frequency of seizures and psychiatric
disturbance. Other studies provide contradictory evidence.
Dodrill (1981a), for example, noted a clear association between
the lifetime number of seizures and the severity of psychopathology. However, Dodrill's research involved adults, suggesting that
it may take several years before the relationship between seizure
frequency and psychopathology becomes manifest.

TREATMENT

ANTI-CONVULSANT MEDICATIONS

Without question, anti-convulsant medications have been the
most beneficial treatment for seizures. Bromides, which were used
previously, had widespread side effects (Livingston, 1966).
Bromide medications were replaced in the early part of this

century with phenobarbital, and somewhat later with phenytoin ("Epilepsy," 1980). However, these drugs were not without side effects, and because they were ineffective for certain seizure types, a variety of additional anticonvulsant medications were developed ("Epilepsy," 1980). The NINCDS Epilepsy Branch ("Epilepsy," 1980) has documented 16 anti-convulsant drugs that are currently marketed, of which the three newest medications are carbamazepine (Tegretol), clonazepam (Clonopin), and valproic acid (Depakene). Table 3 lists the most commonly used anti-convulsant medications, the seizure types for which they are generally pre-scribed, and their common side effects.

Nearly half of epileptics become seizure-free and an addi-tional 25% receive significant relief from seizures after adminis-tration of anti-convulsant medication (Thomas, & Knotts, 1976). Numerous factors contribute to the successful control of seizures by anti-convulsant medication. These include increased sophisti-cation in identifying the seizure type (Penry & Newmark, 1979), new and more effective drugs ("Epilepsy," 1980), and improved methods for determining serum anticonvulsant blood levels (Dodson et al., 1976a). The effectiveness of drug therapy depends upon a successful match between specific type of anti-convulsant and sei-zure type (Penry & Newmark, 1979). Livingston (1966) reports that phenobarbital is especially effective in controlling grand mal seizures. Interestingly, children may require higher doses of phenobarbital per kilogram of body weight than adults in order to achieve the desired anti-convulsant effect (Livingston, 1966). The benefits of anti-convulsants are also related to the severity of the seizure disorder. Patients who have several episodes each day are generally less responsive to drug regimens (Penry & Newmark, 1979).

Drug side effects. All of the medications discussed in the previous section have been shown to control or reduce seizures successfully. However, each drug produces side effects, some of which can seriously impair functioning on a short-term, and pos-sibly on a permanent, basis as well (Dreifuss, 1975). Phenobarb-ital produces psychomotor slowing (Hutt et al., 1968), and impairs performance on numerous neuropsychological measures (Hartlage, 1981). Marchesi (1979) reports that vigilance is attenuated after administration of phenobarbital, primidone, or phenytoin. Memory capacities improve after phenobarbital or primidone dosages are reduced, although the number of seizures accordingly increases (Oxley, 1979).

Trimble (1979a) found a relationship between children's dis-ruptive behavior and several anti-convulsant medications, includ-ing phenobarbital, primidone, and phenytoin. Dreifuss (1975) re-ported that hyperactivity may be manifest after certain anti-con-vulsant drugs are administered. Viukari et al. (1972) observed low serum calcium levels in mentally subnormal epileptics who were receiving phenytoin anti-convulsant drug therapy. Higher blood levels of certain anti-convulsants, such as sulthiame and pheny- toin, occur in persons with low IQs (Trimble, 1979b). Patients receiving high therapeutic doses of diphenyhydantoin perform more poorly on motor tasks than patients who are administered lower doses (Reynolds & Travers, 1974; Dodrill, 1975). Although Dodson et al. (1976a) report "remarkably few" side effects from valproic acid, recently this drug has been found to result in diminished production of blood proteins in the liver ("Drug Side Effects," 1980).

New techniques for monitoring serum anti-convulsant levels, such as gas liquid chromatography, have greatly enhanced our capacity to study the side effects of seizure control medications (Dodson et al., 1976a; "Epilepsy," 1980). These procedures also are useful for monitoring individual patients so that toxic levels of medication are not attained (Dodson et al., 1976a). Hartlage (1981) reported that scores on the Digit Symbol, Coding, and Finger Oscillation tests were negatively correlated with serum anti-convulsant levels of phenobarbital and primidone. Within the therapeutic range for phenobarbital, test performance was associ- ated with serum anti-convulsant level (Hartlage, 1981). These findings indicate that even within therapeutic levels of anti-con- vulsant medications, there may be impaired cognitive functioning. Similarly, MacLeod et al. (1978) demonstrated that short-term memory was disrupted at higher serum levels on phenobarbital. Long-term memory, however, was not affected. Although both of these studies examined adults, the findings nonetheless have im- plications for children who have seizure disorders that are being treated with phenobarbital (MacLeod et al., 1978).

While few clinicians would deny the general effectiveness of anticonvulsant medications, it is evident that the long-term administration of such drugs does not occur without some physio- logical or psychological cost to the patient. Nevertheless, despite such cost, it is preferable in nearly all cases to control prolonged seizure activity (Dodrill, 1981a). With the capacity to monitor drug levels in the blood, toxic levels of medications can be prevented. However, it is important to emphasize that even therapeutic levels of some anti-convulsant drugs are associated with depressed performance on certain types of tasks (MacLeod et al., 1978; Hartlage, 1981).

NONPHARMACOLOGICAL INTERVENTIONS

The majority of nonmedical interventions do not have neuro- psychological ramifications, nor are they used extensively with children. Hence, they will be discussed only briefly. One example of a nonpharmacological treatment is the ketogenic diets which comprise a fat/nonfat ratio of 3:1 to 4:1. The effectiveness of the ketogenic diet has been demonstrated both as a sole treatment and when used in conjunction with anti-convulsant medications (Dodson et al., 1976b). The ketogenic diet is especially recommended in cases where drug toxicity levels are a factor (Dodson et al., 1976b). Other nonpharmacological therapies include behavioral modification, such as biofeedback (Cott et al., 1979), and reinforcement contingency programs (Mostofsky & Balaschak, 1977).

SURGERY

No intervention is more controversial than the use of surgery (Smith, & Kiloh, 1977). This practice is reminiscent of 18th century trephining (Temkin, 1971), and of the widespread practice in this century of performing psychosurgery to control behavioral disorders such as aggression and sexual aberrations, as well as various psychopathological disturbances (Smith & Kiloh, 1977).

Despite the negative connotations, surgery often is successful in cases of intractable epilepsy (Falconer, 1974; Dodson et al., 1976b; Taylor, 1976; Kiloh, 1977; "Epilepsy," 1980). Uncontrollable seizures often occur where there is an epileptogenic focus due to scar tissue (Polkey, 1976). In such cases, excision of superficial cortical scars may be recommended (Taylor, 1976). Falconer (1974) reports follow-up results for 30 children who were treated surgically for intractable temporal lobe epilepsy. Sixty percent of the children were seizure-free following surgery, and 40% showed lesser improvement. The surgery was successful on children as young as five or six years of age. Falconer advocates surgery as the treatment of choice for temporal lobe epilepsy that cannot be controlled by anti-convulsant medications.

Dodson et al. (1976b) adopt a somewhat more cautious viewpoint, arguing that it is advisable to delay surgery for several years in patients with intractable seizures. They suggest that this is prudent because new anti-convulsant drugs may become available that could provide relief. They also emphasize that seizures often change with age, and may even disappear altogether. Despite their caveats, Dodson et al. (1976b) have performed surgery on children with uncontrollable seizures and have reported the outcome for nine children. Five of the children have had substantially fewer seizures, and three of the five have been seizure-free. The follow-up period for two of the patients was too brief for an unequivocal conclusion about outcome, although these children at the time of the report were currently without seizures. Two of the nine patients were unchanged after the surgery. None of the nine children suffered neurological deterioration or impairments from the surgery. These results, though on a small sample, are promising, and suggest that surgical intervention can be effective.

Neuropsychological testing, employing techniques advanced by Wada and Rasmussen (1960), can provide useful information for determining the advisability of surgery for a given patient. This procedure, routinely employed in some neuro-surgical settings, involves alternately injecting sodium amytal into the left and right internal carotid arteries. During the period of sedation produced by the sodium amytal, a systematic neuropsychological assessment can be conducted to determine the lateralization and localization of psychological functions. Subsequently, in patients found appropriate for resection, especially those for whom the surgical procedure involves the hemisphere dominant for speech, intraoperative neuropsychological testing can help localize critical cortical areas which must be spared to enable the patient to retain necessary cognitive abilities (Hartlage & Flanigin, 1982).

SUMMARY

The condition of childhood epilepsy is associated with a wide range of neuropsychological phenomena of relevance for research and treatment. Although many studies concerning intellectual characteristics of children with epilepsy report subnormal functioning, further investigation of these findings is desirable. Until recently, many children with epilepsy were excluded from regular classrooms, which may have depressed intellectual performance scores. Furthermore, since the introduction of more effective anti-convulsant medications, greater numbers of children are able to have their seizures controlled, and this reduction in seizure activity may be directly related to mitigation of intellectual deterioration. Finally, the introduction of advanced techniques for the purpose of monitoring serum anti-convulsant levels permits researchers to carefully evaluate the specific effects of various doses of individual anti-convulsants in ways which relate to a wide range of neuropsychological behaviors, such as vigilance, attention, memory, and sensory and motor integrity.

In addition to the effects of epilepsy and various treatment approaches on mental development characteristics of children, psychological and behavioral aspects are also of critical importance. In the past, much attention has been directed toward the dynamic variables related to specific behavioral characteristics of persons with epilepsy. While certainly any chronic illness is associated with a certain degree of psychological adjustment problems, recently emphasis has been redirected to the physiological etiology of such symptomatology in epileptic populations. While such research has only begun, much of this work suggests that a specific seizure focus may be directly translated into affective behavior. More research into the various manners of expression of specific neurological disorders can assist the psychologist in preparing the epileptic child, as well as parents and teachers, for subsequent behavioral phenomena.

REFERENCES

Ajmone-Marson, C., & Ralston, B.L. **The epileptic seizure. Its functional morphology and diagnostic significance.** Springfield, Ill: Charles C. Thomas, 1957.

Andermann, E. Genetic factors explored. **National Spokesman,** 1979, 12, 6.

Ansbaugh, D.J., Gilliland, M., & Ansbaugh, S.J. The student with epilepsy. **Today's Education,** 1980, 69, 78E-86E.

Bagley, C. **The social psychology of the epileptic child.** Coral Gables, Fla: University of Miami Press, 1971.

Batzel, L.W., Dodrill, C.B., & Fraser, R.T. Further validation of the WPSI vocational scale: Comparison with other correlates of employment in epilepsy. **Epilepsia,** 1980, 21, 235-242.

Boll, T.J. Conceptual vs. perceptual vs. motor deficits in brain-damaged children. **Journal of Clinical Psychology,** 1972, 28, 157-159.

Boll, T.J., Richards, H., & Berent, S. Tactile-perceptual functioning and academic performance in brain-impaired and un-impaired children. **Perceptual and Motor Skills,** 1978, 47, 491-495.

Carlberg, C. & Kavale, K. The efficacy of special versus regular class placement for exceptional children: A meta-analysis. **Journal of Special Education,** 1980, 14, 295-309.

Cooper, J.A. & Ferry, P.C. Acquired auditory verbal agnosia and seizures in childhood. **Journal of Speech and Hearing Disorders,** 1978, 43, 176-184.

Cott, A., Pavloski, R.P., & Block, A.H. Reducing epileptic seizures through operant conditioning of central nervous system activity: Procedural variables. **Science,** 1979, 203, 73-75.

Dean, R.S. Total seizure estimate as a predictor of cognitive variables with children. **Clinical Neuropsychology,** in press.

Dennerll, R.D., Broeder, J.D., & Sokolov, S.L. WISC and WAIS factors in children and adults with epilepsy. **Journal of Clinical Psychology,** 1964, 20, 236-240.

Dodrill, C.B. Diphenylhydantoin serum levels, toxicity, and neuropsychological performance in patients with epilepsy. **Epilepsia,** 1975, 16, 593-600.

Dodrill, C.B. Interrelationships between neuropsychological data and social problems in epilepsy. In R. Canger, F. Angeleri, & J.R. Penry (Eds.), **Advances in epileptology: XIth Epilepsy International Symposium.** New York: Raven Press, 1980.

Dodrill, C.B. Effects of major motor seizures upon neuropsychological and emotional functioning. In J.T. Marsh (Chair),

Neuropsychology and psychopathology. Paper presented at the meeting of the American Psychological Association, Los Angeles, 1981a.

Dodrill, C.B., Batzel, L.W., Queisser, H.R., & Temkin, N.R. An objective method for the assessment of psychological and social problems among epileptics. **Epilepsia,** 1980, 21, 123–135.

Dodson, W.E., Prensky, A.L., DeVivo, D.C., Goldring, S., & Dodge, P.R. Management of seizure disorders: Selected aspects, Part I. **The Journal of Pediatrics,** 1976a, **89,** 527–540.

Dodson, W.E., Prensky, A.L., DeVivo, D.C., Goldring, S., & Dodge, P.R. Management of seizures disorders: Selected aspects, Part II. **The Journal of Pediatrics,** 1976b, **89,** 695–703.

Dreifuss, F.E. The nature of epilepsy. In G.H. Wright (Ed.), **Epilepsy rehabilitation.** Boston: Little, Brown, & Co., 1975.

Droose, H. Genetic factors explored. **National Spokesman,** 1979, 12, 6.

Drug side effects. **USA Today,** 1980, 105, 15.

Epilepsy, the NINCDS research program. Bethesda, MD: National Institutes of Health, 1980.

Falconer, M.A. Mesial temporal (Ammon's horn) sclerosis as a common cause of epilepsy—aetiology, treatment, and prevention. **The Lancet,** 1974, 2, 767–770.

Fedio, P. & Mirsky, A.F. Selective intellectual deficits in children with temporal lobe or centracephalic epilepsy. **Neuropsychologia,** 1969, 7, 287–300.

Forster, F.M. **Reflex epilepsy, behavioral therapy and conditional reflexes.** Springfield, IL: Charles C. Thomas, 1977.

Gastaut, H. **Inquiry into the education of epileptic children.** Paper presented at the second seminar of the International Bureau for Epilepsy, Marseilles, 1964.

Geschwind, N., Shader, R.I., Bear, D., North, B., Levin, K., & Chetham, D. Behavioral changes with temporal lobe epilepsy: Assessment and treatment. **Journal of Clinical Psychiatry,** 1980, **41,** 89–95.

Gilmore, R.L. & Heilman, R.M. Speech arrest in partial seizures: Evidence of an associated language disorder. **Neurology,** 1981, **31,** 1016–1019.

Goldin, G.J., Perry, S.L., Margolin, R.J., Statsky, B.A., & Foster, J.C. **The rehabilitation of the young epileptic.** Lexington, MA: D.C. Heath & Co., 1971.

Green, J.B. & Hartlage, L.C. Comparative performance of epileptic and nonepileptic children and adolescents. **Diseases of the Nervous System,** 1971, 32, 418–421.

Halstead, H. Abilities and behavior of epileptic children. **Journal of Mental Science,** 1957, 103, 28–47.

Harris, P. Clinical and biochemical aspects of epilepsy. In H.F. Bradford & C.D. Marsden (Eds.), **Biochemistry and neurology.** London: Academic Press, 1976.

Hartlage, L.C. Neuropsychological assessment of anti-convulsant drug toxicity. **Clinical neuropsychology**, 1981, 3,

Hartlage, L.C. & Flanigin, H. Neuropsychological aspects of temporal lobe resection in epilepsy. **Clinical Neuropsychology**, 1982, 4, 89-90.

Hartlage, L.C. & Green, J.B. The EEG as a predictor of intellective and academic performance. **Journal of Learning Disabilities**, 1973, 6, 239-242.

Hauser, W.A. & Kurland, L.T. Incidence, prevalence, time trends of convulsive disorders in Rochester, Minnesota: A community survey. In M. Alter, & W.A. Hauser (Eds.), **The epidemiology of epilepsy.** Washington, D.C.: Department of Health, Education and Welfare, 1972.

Hedgeman, B.S. Epilepsy action for reducing barriers to employment and community participation. In L.G. Perlman (Ed.), **The role of vocational rehabilitation in the 1980's.** Washington, D.C.: National Rehabilitation Association, 1978.

Hermann, B.P. Psychological effects of epilepsy: A review. **Catalog of Selected Documents in Psychology**, 1977, 7, 17.

Hughes, J.R. & Olson, S.F. An investigation of eight different types of temporal lobe discharges. **Epilepsia**, 1981, 22, 421-435.

Hutt, S.J., Jackson, P.M., Belsham, A., & Higgins, G. Perceptual-motor behavior in relation to blood phenobarbitone level: A preliminary report. **Developmental Medicine and Child Neurology**, 1968, 10, 626-632.

Ives, L.A. Learning difficulties in children with epilepsy. **British Journal of Disorders of Communication**, 1970, 5, 77-84.

Jeavons, P.M. **Hospital update**, January, 1975, 11-22.

Kaufman, A.S. WISC-R research: Implications for interpretation. **School Psychology Digest**, 1979, 8, 5-27.

Kaufman, D.M. **Clinical neurology for psychiatrists.** New York: Grune & Stratton, 1981.

Kiloh, L.G. The treatment of anger and aggression and the modification of sexual deviation. In J.S. Smith, & L.G. Kiloh (Eds.), **Psychosurgery and society.** New York: Pergaman Press, 1977.

King, D.W., Gallagher, B.B., Murvin, A.J., Smith, D.B., Marcus, D.J., Hartlage, L.C., & Ward, L.C. Pseudo seizures: Diagnostic evaluation. **Neurology**, 1982, 32, 18-23.

Levine, D.N., Hier, D.B., & Calvanio, R. Acquired learning disability for reading after left temporal lobe damage in childhood. **Neurology**, 1981, 31, 257-264.

Lezak, M.D. **Neuropsychological assessment.** New York: Oxford University Press, 1976.

Lisansky, E.S. Convulsive disorders and personality. **Journal of Abnormal and Social Psychology**, 1948, 20, 29-37.

Livingston, S. **Drug therapy for epilepsy.** Springfield, IL: Charles C. Thomas, 1966.

MacLeod, C.M., Dekaban, A., & Hunt, E. Memory impairment in epileptic patients: Selective effects of phenobarbital concentration. **Science**, 1978, **202**, 1102–1104.

Marchesi, G.F. Drugs and brain function. **National Spokesman**, 1979, 12, 6.

Metrakos, J.D. & Matrakos, K. Genetics of convulsive disorders. I. Introduction problems, methods, and baselines. **Neurology**, 1960, 10, 228–240.

Millikan, C.H. **Seizure disorder: Diagnosis.** Detroit: Parke-Davis, 1976 (1975?).

Mostofsky, D.I. & Balaschak, B.A. Psychobiological control of seizures. **Psychological Bulletin**, 1977, 84, 723–750.

Nuffield, E.J.A. Neurophysiology and behavior disorders in epileptic children. **Journal of Mental Science**, 1961, 107, 438–458.

Ounsted, C. The hyperkinetic syndrome in epileptic children. **The Lancet**, 1955, 303.

Oxley, J. Drugs and brain function. **National Spokesman**, 1979, 12, 7.

Penry, J.K., & Newmark, M.E. The use of antiepileptic drugs. **Annals of Internal Medicine**, 1979, **90**, 207–218.

Plan for nationwide action on epilepsy. Vol. 1. Washington, D.C.: U.S. Department of Health, Education and Welfare, 1977.

Polkey, C.E. Lesions in human epilepsy. In H.F. Bradford, & C.D. Marsden (Eds.), **Biochemistry and neurology.** London: Academic Press, 1976.

Pond, D.A. Psychiatric aspects of epileptic and brain-damaged children. **British Medical Journal**, 1961, 1, 377–382.

Pond, D.A. & Bidwell, B.H. A survey of epilepsy in fourteen general practices II. Social and psychological aspects. **Epilepsia**, 1960, 1, 285–299.

Reynolds, E.H. & Travers, R.D. Serum anti-convulsant concentration in epileptic patients with mental symptoms. **British Journal of Psychiatry**, 1974, 124, 440–445.

Ritchie, K. Research note: Interactions in the families of epileptic children. **Journal of Child Psychology and Psychiatry and Allied Disciplines**, 1981, 22, 65–71.

Robb, J.P. A review of epidemiologic concepts of epilepsy. In M. Alter, & W.A. Hausser (Eds.), **The epidemiology of epilepsy.** (NINDS Monograph No. 14). Washington, D.C.: U.S. Department of Health, Education and Welfare, 1972.

Rodin, E.A. Medical considerations. In G.N. Wright (Ed.), **Epilepsy rehabilitation.** Boston: Little, Brown and Company, 1975.

Rutter, M., Graham, P., & Yule, W. **A neuropsychiatric study in childhood.** Philadelphia: J.B. Lippincott Co., 1970.

Seidenberg, M., O'Leary, D.S., Berent, S., & Boll, T. Changes in seizure frequency and test-retest scores on the Wechsler Adult Intelligence Test. **Epilepsia**, 1981, 22, 75–83.

Smith, J.S. & Kiloh, L.G.   Introduction.   In J.S. Smith & L.G. Kiloh (Eds.), **Psychosurgery and society.** New York: Pergaman Press, 1977.

Stores, G., Hart, J., & Piran, N.   Inattentiveness in school children with epilepsy. **Epilepsia**, 1978, 19, 169–175.

Taylor, D.C.   Developmental stratagems organizing intellectual skills: Evidence from studies temporal lobectomy for epilepsy.   In R.M. Knights & D.J. Bakker (Eds.), **The neuropsychology of learning disorders.** Baltimore: University Park Press, 1976.

Temkin, O. **The falling sickness** (2nd ed.).   Baltimore: The Johns Hopkins Press, 1971.

Thomas, J.A. & Knotts, G.R.   Epilepsy and other seizure disorders in children: Drug management. **The Journal of School Health,** 1976, 46, 462–465.

Tizzard, B.   The personality of epileptics: A discussion of the evidence. **Psychological Bulletin,** 1962, 59, 196–210.

Townsend, H.R.A.   Epilepsy – a clinician's view. In H.F. Bradford & C.D. Marsden (Eds.), **Biochemistry and neurology.** London: Academic Press, 1976.

Trimble, M.   Drugs and behavior. **National Spokesman,** 1979a, 12, 6.

Trimble, M.   Drugs and I.Q. **National Spokesman,** 1979b, 12, 7.

Viukari, N.M.A., Tammisto, P., & Kauko, K.   Low serum calcium levels in forty mentally subnormal epileptics. **Journal of Mental Deficiency Research,** 1972, 16, 192–195.

Vogel, W. & Broverman, D.M.   Relationship between EEG and test intelligence: A critical review. **Psychological Bulletin,** 1964, 62, 132–144.

Wada, J. & Rasmussen, T.   Intracarotid injection of sodium amytal for the lateralization of cerebral dominance. **Journal of Neurosurgery,** 1960, 17, 266–282.

Watts, G.O. **Dynamic neuro–science: Its application to brain disorders.** Hagerstown, MD: Harper & Row, 1975.

Williams, M. **Brain damage, behaviour, and the mind.** New York: John Wiley & Sons, 1979.

Wright, G.N.   Rehabilitation and the problem of epilepsy.   In G.N. Wright (Ed.), **Epilepsy rehabilitation.** Boston: Little, Brown and Company, 1975.

DYSLEXIA

Harold W. Gordon

Department of Psychiatry
University of Pittsburgh School of Medicine
Pittsburgh, Pennsylvania

The perennial puzzle of a child who reads poorly despite normal intellect and absence of diseases beyond chicken pox and the common cold still defies solution. Dyslexic children have been described, diagnosed, characterized, labeled, classified, and reclassified by educators, pediatricians, neurologists, social scientists, psychologists, educational psychologists, social psychologists, school psychologists, testing psychologists, clinical psychologists, psychiatric psychologists, and finally, neuropsychologists. The unique ways in which these individuals perform are well-documented, yet the problem persists. The most serious consequence of this diversity is the multitude of treatments, remedial training, behavior modification, and medications that are developed to deal with these individuals. Successes have been claimed for all, yet newer techniques are continually being developed and marketed as the process is perpetuated. One gets the impression that virtually every method effects an improvement, yet none works well (or well enough). Thus, more research is deemed necessary, producing even more techniques in a seemingly unending and costly spiral.

We make no claims in this chapter to halt the spiral nor to give the final answer, or to give insight where others have failed. However, we do provide a new perspective that accounts for previous data. In a sense, our approach is radical in that we start with a bias rather than an open mind; we conclude that our bias is correct and the next step is to proceed from there. The origin of the bias is an informal observation in the dyslexia clinic that difficulties in sequential processing are associated with reading and other learning difficulties, while more perceptual or patterned tasks are performed normally. The observation is, of course, well known and has been reported in a number of contexts. Our bias extends the observation to the conjecture that reading disabled children perform below average on tasks usually attributed to the left cerebral hemisphere but perform at least normally on tasks usually associated with the right hemisphere. It should be mentioned that we include only those reading disabled individuals who fulfill the narrow definition by exclusion: reading difficulties without abnormally low IQ's, no "hard" neurological deficits or physical handicaps, appropriate environment stimulation and learning opportunities. We suggest that the asymmetry would arise not from poor language performance, per se, but rather from basic left hemisphere dysfunction under-lying a number of processes, of which language is one. Before data are presented in support of this hypothesis, however, a brief critique of other approaches is in order.

PSYCHOLOGICAL TESTS, ACHIEVEMENT TESTS, AND READING ABILITY

Several studies have attempted to predict learning disabil-ities in children on the basis of psychological tests (intelli-gence, aptitude, and achievement), given in early grades, as an indication of performance on reading or other tests of achieve-ment, given later. These studies achieve success inasmuch as they correctly select the extremes: those at high risk for disability as well as those not at risk. The studies differ on 1) the rela-tive size of the false positive and false negative subgroups, and 2) the convenience of the test instrument for practical use in screening and assessment.

In one study (Ferinden & Jacobson, 1970), a standard achieve-ment test (the Wide Range Achievement Test) and a subjective test of figure drawing (Evanston Early Identification Scale) were ac-curate in selecting children with potential learning disabili-ties. The Metropolitan Reading Test predicted only at the ex-tremes; the Bender-Gestalt Visual Motor Test was no help whatso-ever—a theme that repeated itself in other perceptual-motor tests (e.g., Husak & Magill, 1979). In a similar study (Serwer, Shapiro, & Shapiro, 1972), aptitude measures of numerical ability from both the Primary Mental Abilities and Metropolitan Readiness Test were also good indicators but, again, kindergarten teachers were nearly as successful. On the other hand, subtests of the WISC, PMA, ITPA, Detroit tests, and Frostig had little or no cor-relation with the Metropolitan Achievement Test administered later. The same negative finding was reported for the PMA and some visuomotor tasks by another study attempting to assess kin-dergarten children at risk (Badian & Serwer, 1975).

Finally, in following up children who had been assessed on both a developmental test (Denver Developmental Screening Test) and an IQ test (Stanford-Binet), 30% of the children found to be

normal on one of the tests nevertheless developed school problems
(Camp, Van Doornick, Frankenburg, & Lampe, 1977). Furthermore,
25% of the subjects who had low IQ's and questionable or abnormal
developmental scores turned out to have no school problems. In
summary, teachers are often as accurate in designating children
who will have learning disabilities as are aptitude, intelligence,
and some developmental tests, thus emphasizing the failure of this
approach to give clear direction for understanding the basis of
learning disabilities.

NEUROPSYCHOLOGICAL VARIABLES AND READING ACHIEVEMENT

Since aptitude, intelligence, and achievement tests draw upon
a relatively large number of basic cognitive functions, failure of
these measures to be better predictors may be related to the complexity of the variables. That is, each test would measure a number of different cognitive functions. The approach of neuropsychology is to counter this problem. Tests are chosen which are
designed to assess functions of the brain more "basic" or unidi-
mensional in their scope (Mattis, French, & Rapin, 1975; Rourke &
Orr, 1977; Doehring & Hoshko, 1977; Fletcher & Satz, 1980). One
study showed that search and recognition of a complex geometric
figure, or a sequence of geometric figures was predictive of reading success in reading disabled children but not in normal readers
(Rourke & Orr, 1977). Similar tests in the same battery, using
letters instead of geometric forms, were *poorer* predictors, suggesting that the verbal nature of the stimuli is *not* the critical
factor for picking up reading problems.

In a large longitudinal study covering the early school
years, Kindergarten to Grade five, thirteen neuropsychological
test variables were presented to nearly five hundred children
(Fletcher & Satz, 1980). A factor analysis produced three major
factors--none of which, alone, were predictive of reading difficulties: Spatial/perceptual tests best predicted longitudinal
achievement; verbal tests best predicted concurrent achievement.
In establishing predictor variables (Satz, Taylor, Friel, &
Fletcher, 1978), the percentage of correct predictions was in the
80's for the extreme cases while only 2/3 of the milder cases of
disabilities were correctly predicted. The best one can say is
that manifestation of school achievement difficulties is complex
and represents the intersection of neuropsychological factors with
other factors. What is unfortunate is that neither the predictor
variables, factors, nor the few tests that discriminated well provided a good theory as to the underlying, brain-related features
that may cause learning disabilities. It was for this reason neuropsychological testing was instituted in the first place.

In a different approach, reading disabled children were carefully identified *a priori* according to standard criteria. By ad-

ministering neuropsychological tests to this group, it was hoped
that common neuropsychological characteristics could be identified
(Haring & Ridgway, 1967; Farrar & Leigh, 1972). The results were
unsuccessful, possibly because the tests were inappropriate or the
definition of reading disability was self-limiting.

Reading disabilities need not be mutually exclusive of other
disorders; on the contrary, a number of disorders may well occur
together. Similarly, certain cognitive factors associated with
reading ability may not sufficiently determine presence or absence
of disabilities. These points are well documented by a study
(Taylor, Satz, & Friel, 1979) in which "dyslexic" disabled readers
were distinguished from "non-dyslexic" disabled readers if they
had one or more of the following: 1) a picture vocabulary IQ
greater than 90; 2) average or above socioeconomic status; and, 3)
absence of emotional, sensory, or neurological symptomatology.
Nevertheless, there were no differences between these groups on
factors of 1) severity of reading difficulty, 2) letter reversals,
3) disorders in other academic areas, 4) parent reading disabilities, 5) neurological abnormalities, 6) neuropsychological performance and 7) personality traits. These studies suggest that *a
priori* selection of reading disabled children will not necessarily
help in discovering underlying features.

TOWARD A COGNITIVE PROFILE FOR READING DISABLED CHILDREN

In the midst of failures to find consistent psychological
constructs for children with reading disabilities, a number of
studies have pointed out some regularities in observations. One
important contribution has been the operational classification of
children according to spelling errors (Boder, 1973). Children
were divided into 3 groups according to whether words in the
child's sight vocabulary 1) bore no relation to the sound of the
word ("dysphonetic" subjects), 2) were fair phonetic approxima-
tions of the word ("dyseidetic" subjects), or 3) had errors that
were the combination of the two. While the description of these
children stopped short of comparison to left or right hemisphere
function, dysphonetic children would appear to have dysfunction
more closely associated with processes in the left hemisphere and
dyseidetic children would appear to have right hemisphere
deficits.

Another observation relevant to the hemispheric contribution
to reading disabilities, is the deficiency of such children in
phonological decoding (Vellutino, 1978). More importantly, it is
the distinction between acoustic processing, which reading disabled children may be able to do, and phonetic or lingusitic decoding, which they cannot do, that is critical (Liberman, Shankweiler, Fischer, & Carter, 1974). Whereas both hemispheres may

decode acoustically, it is probably only the left that can decode linguistically (Zaidel, 1978).

In further support of what appears to be a left hemisphere deficiency relative to right is a consistent observation that Performance IQ is higher than Verbal IQ. In one study of 56 reading disabled children (Naidoo, 1972), twice as many children had greater Performance IQ's than Verbal IQ's, in spite of the fact that the Digit Span subtest (the most sequential and typcially the most difficult test for dyslexics) was not used in the calculation of the Verbal IQ. The Digit Span was the worst test (scaled score = 8.3) and was four points lower (1.3 standard deviations) than performance on the Block Design, the best test. Essentially the same discrepancy between Digit Span and Block Design was seen in another group of forty-one spelling "retardates" from the same series.

In a review of twenty-one studies including more than 1350 children (Rugel, 1974), the performance on the Digit Span was again below Block Design and Object Assembly in nineteen of the studies, and below Picture Completion in all of them. The (weighted) average difference between Digit Span and these three subtests was statistically enormous: nearly 1.0 standard deviation (2.5 scaled points). When the WISC subtests from each of the same 21 studies were regrouped into three categories, *Spatial* (Object Assembly, Block Design, and Picture Completion), *Sequential* (Digit Span, Picture Arrangement and Coding), and *Conceptual* (Comprehension, Similarities, and Vocabulary), the Spatial category was performed the best in 80% of the studies, and it was always performed better than the Sequential category. Similar asymmetries were obtained in other samples of school-labeled "learning disabled" children (Smith, Coleman, Dokecki, & Davis, 1977).

The significance of these WISC studies is that the Digit Span has an important sequential component and is associated with left hemisphere function. Block Design and Object Assembly have a perceptual or constructional component and are associated with right hemisphere function (Parsons, Vega, & Burn, 1968; Bentin & Gordon, 1979). Poor sequential ability as exhibited by poor performance on the Digit Span is well known in reading disabled children (Bakker, 1967) and supports the notion that there are deficits in functioning or development (Satz & Sparrow, 1970) of the left cerebral hemisphere. By contrast, relatively good performances on Block Design, Object Assembly and other visuo-spatial tasks suggest at least normal functioning in tests attributed to the right cerebral hemisphere (Benton, 1975).

Based on these same observations that specific cognitive characteristics typically accompany children with learning disabilities, an experimental approach anticipating our own was attempted in which children were selected on the basis of Low Verbal/High Performance scores on the WISC (Richman & Lindgren, 1980). Noting that others had failed in this approach presumably because they had selected subjects from a learning disabled population, the new approach selected children from a pediatric psychology outpatient unit who were *unselected* for learning disability. Even though the results of the study confirmed that learning disabled children had a different cognitive organization than normal children, it failed to support the premise on which it was based; namely, that learning-disabled children were poor at sequential abilities. One of the explanations for this discrepancy was that the subtests of the WISC may not have been appropriate in differentiating subjects. Their choice of test instruments was motivated by a desire for a measure of intellectual ability that required verbal mediation but not verbal comprehension or a verbal response. We would agree that the choice of tests is critical and have based our selection, in part, on the theoretical framework that the "asymmetrical" cognitive organization observed in learning-disabled children is related to an asymmetry of cognitive processes attributed to the left and right hemispheres of the brain (Kaufman, 1979).

The Dichotomy of Function in the Right and Left Hemispheres

The separation of cognitive processes into the left and right hemispheres proposed in the last century by Jackson (Jackson, 1874) has been validated over the years. The left hemisphere has been considered dominant for speech and other language functions dating from as far back as the early phrenologists (Combe, 1843). The different functions attributed to the right hemisphere have been determined much more slowly, starting with the observation that constructional apraxia occurred more often in patients with right hemisphere lesions (Patterson & Zangwill, 1944; Zangwill, 1960; Piercy & Smythe, 1962).

Empirical investigations have demonstrated right hemisphere superiority in three areas: 1) form or pattern perception; 2) orientation in space; and, 3) localization in space. Right dominance for pattern perception has been inferred from poor performances by patients with right hemisphere lesions in recognition of nonsense shapes (De Renzi, Faglioni, & Scotti, 1968; De Renzi & Scotti, 1969). Positive evidence in patients with complete forebrain commissurotomy has confirmed the right hemisphere superiority for tactual or visual shape perception (Bogen & Gazzaniga, 1965; Milner & Taylor, 1972; Levy, Trevarthen, & Sperry, 1972; Zaidel & Sperry, 1973; Franco & Sperry, 1977) and closure (Nebes, 1971; Nebes, 1972; Bogen, De Zure, Ten Houten, & Marsh, 1972), as has similar evidence in neurologically intact subjects (Rizzolatti, Umilta, & Berlucci, 1971; Geffen, Bradshaw, &

Wallace, 1971; Cohen, 1973; Witelson, 1974; Umilta, Bagnara, & Simion, 1978; Ornstein, Johnstone, Herron, & Swencionis, 1980).

Spatial orientation has been attributed to the parietal area of both hemispheres (Butters & Barton, 1970), but deficits in patients with right lesions for accurately perceiving the directionality, both visually and tactually for a rod (De Renzi, Faglioni, & Scotti, 1971), manikin figures (Ratcliff, 1979), line segments (Warrington & Rabin, 1970; Benton, Hannay, & Varney, 1975), and directions of movement (Carmon & Benton, 1969; Fountenot & Benton, 1971) imply right hemisphere superiority. Positive evidence of right hemisphere superority has also been shown for line directionality in intact subjects (Fountenot & Benton, 1972; Benton, Levin, & Varney, 1973; Umilta, Rizzolatti, Marzi, Zamboni, Franzini, Camardo, & Berlucchi, 1974). Electroencephalographic measures of alpha ratios that theoretically show relative cerebral activity have provided mixed results, but significant correlations have been shown between level of performance in a complex rotation task and degree of right hemisphere involvement (Ornstein et al., 1980; Furst, 1976). Finally, deficits for locating points in space either visually or tactually have been shown in patients with right hemisphere lesions (Faglioni, Scotti, & Spinnler) while right hemisphere dominance has been confirmed in intact subjects (Kimura, 1969; Levy & Reid, 1976), although this has been disputed (Bryden, 1976).

Language, speech in particular, is the dominant cognitive function of the left hemisphere even though comprehension abilities are also found for the right hemisphere (Zaidel, 1978). But in addition, temporality or sequencing has been attributed to the left hemisphere. Left dominance was implied from deficits in aphasics for the judgement of simultaneity (Efron, 1963) and for the perception of temporal ordering in non-aphasic patients with left hemisphere lesions (Carmon & Nachshon, 1971). Deficits in sequential processing are also found in developmental dyslexics (Gordon, 1980) and developmental dysphasics (Tallal & Piercy, 1973). Left hemisphere dominance for temporal processing is further confirmed in intact subjects where stimuli were presented temporally (Halperin, Nachshon, & Carmon, 1973) or rhythmically (Gordon, 1978). Visual sequencing also appears to be left hemisphere dominant (Horan, Ashton, & Minto, 1980) although mixed results may indicate the presence of a spatial element as well (De Renzi, Faglioni, & Villa, 1977; Kim, Royer, Bonstelle, & Boller, 1980).

With the bulk of the research behind us, we have a fairly clear idea of what kinds of tasks are performed better by the right hemisphere and which are performed better by the left. Based on these characteristics it is common to observe that some people appear to perform tasks associated with left hemisphere functioning better than they perform tasks associated with the right hemisphere. Others perform tasks associated with right hemisphere functioning better than they perform tasks associated with the left. While the observations may be true, it does not necessarily follow that such people have a dominant, or more active, left hemisphere or a dominate or more active right hemisphere. In fact, attempts to demonstrate this point have failed (Arnt & Berger, 1978). It is too much of a leap to go from research delineating *where* in the normal brain certain functions are located to predict *how* the normal brain will contribute to day-to-day performance of that behavior. A "left hemisphere person", defined as one who performs better on functions attributed to the left hemisphere, may be performing these primarily "left brain" functions from *both* sides of the cerebrum, perhaps at the expense of "right brain" functions. Research on this point is incomplete.

The study of individuals who favor functions attributed to one hemisphere or the other is interesting. Our aim, as has been foreshadowed, is to show that a large proportion of the reading disabled perform right hemisphere functions better than left. This has been achieved by first developing valid methods by which to assess these individuals.

Since there is no standard degree of hemisphericity, the norm has to be determined empirically, much in the same way as the norm had been determined for "intelligence." Accordingly a battery of tests was designed (The Cognitive Laterality Battery) to assess the relative performance between the abilities attributed to the right and left cerebral hemisphere. A cognitive profile is defined as the relation between performance on right hemisphere tests to performance on left hemisphere tests. By definition, a "normal" performance would not favor either hemisphere. As shall be seen, this Battery was used to assess individuals referred for reading disabilities revealing a consistent profile favoring right hemisphere function.

The Cognitive Laterality Battery (CLB) is a series of tests designed to assess the functions just described for the left and right hemispheres. The tests have been standardized, thus allowing the calculation of Z-scores for individual subjects for each of the tests. Left hemisphere function is best characterized by sequential processing and by verbal output. Accordingly, a test called Serial Sounds was devised in which well-known, easily recognizable sounds (e.g., dog, baby, telephone, etc.) are played in sequences of 3, 4, 5, and 6 items in length. The subject's task is to remember the items in the correct serial order. Partial scoring is awarded if only *part* of a sequence is remembered; the more that is remembered in order, the larger the score. Another sequential test uses numbers as stimuli instead of sounds but otherwise is given in the same way. (This is equivalent to Digit

Span, Forward of the WISC.) Verbal production is another characteristic function of the left hemisphere. Accordingly, tests of
word production (or fluency) are included. The subject is
required to write down as many words as possible that begin with a
given letter of the alphabet. Alternatively, the subject must
write as many words as possible in a given category. Correct
spelling is not required; oral response is allowed, if necessary,
for individually-tested subjects.

Right hemisphere functions are characterized by pattern or
form perception, orientation and spatial localization. Accordingly, point localization is tested by presentation of a large black,
rectangular frame on a white background with an "x" marked some-
where within. The subject's task is to locate (by marking with a
pencil) the corresponding spot on a similar rectangle on an answer
sheet. Orientation is measured by presentation of three 2- or
3-dimensional stimuli. Two of the 3 stimuli are identical but
rotated in space; the third is the mirror image. The subject must
find the two that are identical. Another test presents a stack of
rectangular solids. One of the solids is designated by a number;
the subject must visualize which of the other solids are touching
it. Finally, form perception is assessed by a task of visual
closure in which a form is presented in silhouette with partial
obliteration. The subject must identify the form.

For the purpose of assessing relative hemispheric function,
scores for a subject are converted to Z-scores based on a population mean and standard deviation. A summary score for the right
and left hemispheres, defined as A and P, respectively (named
after the historical terms, "appositional" and "propositional")
(Bogen et al., 1972), are the averages of the appropriate tests.
For the right hemisphere tests A = the average of all Z-scores for
the right hemisphere tests; and, for the left hemisphere P = the
average of all Z-scores of the left hemisphere tests. The cognitive profile, or degree of hemisphericity, is called the Cognitive
Laterality Quotient, CLQ, and is given by the difference between
these measures: CLQ=A-P. Because Z=0 for a "normal" performance
on each of the tests, a "normal" individual will have a theoretical CLQ value of zero. In practice, the distribution of the CLQ
scores centers around zero.

THE COGNITIVE PROFILE OF READING DISABLED CHILDREN

We have observed that reading disabled individuals are more
likely to have difficulties in sequencing and, of course, performing "verbal" tasks while showing at least normal ability on
"visual spatial" or "patterned" tasks. Accordingly, we shall apply the Cognitive Laterality Battery (CLB) to determine the
strength of this observation. The CLB, it will be recalled, is
designed to include tests of functions usually attributed to both

the left and right hemispheres. The applicability of the CLB to the reading disabled population appears to follow since their dichotomy of performance on cognitive tasks resembles the hemisphere dichotomy of cognitive processing. The question is, what will be the profile of an individual referred for reading difficulties in terms of functions normally attributed to the right or left cerebral hemisphere?

The CLB was administered to 150 children referred by teachers, school psychologists or private doctors to a Learning Disability Clinic[1] (Harness, Epstein, & Gordon, 1974). Forty-two of the children are excluded from the analysis because of evidence of "hard" neurological signs, low IQ or apparent cultural deprivation or environmental hardships.

The number of subjects performing better on tests attributed to right hemisphere functioning than on tests of left hemisphere functioning was an overwhelming 97% (105 out of 108). The average difference in performance was more than 1 standard deviation: CLQ=+1.12. This means that the average performance on tests attributed to right hemisphere function was one standard deviation better than performance on tests attributed to left hemisphere function. The distribution of CLQ scores was fairly symmetrical about the mean of 1.12. Only three cases had CLQ's less than zero; three had CLQ's larger that 2.25 (see Figure 1). The distribution

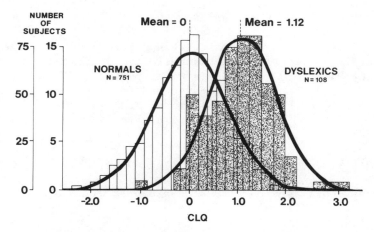

Fig. 1.   Distributions of the CLQ for normal and dyslexic population on the Cognitive Laterality Battery. A normal curve is calculated for each population and superimposed on the distribution.

of CLQ's for a normal population would have similar characteristics but center around CLQ=0 (Figure 1).

The advantage of describing an individual by the *profile* or relationship of test preference—in this case, favoring "visuospatial" functions over "verbal" or "sequential"—rather than *level* of performance is also its disadvantage. Because the CLQ is a *relative* measure, it does not indicate whether the large positive score for the reading disabled subjects is due to poor left hemisphere performance, good right hemisphere performance, or combinations of both. As it happens, the relative performances of the right and left hemispheres of this subject population are rather surprising. The average P — performance on the tests associated with the left cerebral hemisphere — was 0.5 standard deviation *below* average. This, of course, is no surprise since tests of fluency and sequencing required verbal mediation or coding. In either case, the poor results on these tests are consistent with what is generally believed about reading or learning-disabled subjects.

There *is* a surprise in the *above*-average performance on tests attributed to the right hemisphere; the magnitude of superiority was the same 0.5 standard deviation. In other words, *the dyslexic group performed as much above the ability of their peer group on tests of right hemisphere function, as they performed below on tests of left hemisphere function.* The often-seen picture of *failure* on verbal/sequential function is contrasted with *success* on "perceptual," "orientational," or "spatial" function. These findings may clash with one's conception that reading-disabled individuals tend to have perceptual problems, stemming from their reversal of letters or poor performance on the Bender-Gestalt. Part of the inconsistency may be terminology or definition: "perceptual" or "spatial" deficits causing letter reversals may not be qualitatively the same as recognizing a rotation of a two- or three-dimensional object in space. A second reason for the discrepency is that the CLB measurements in the present form are not sensitive to individual variation, precluding the existence of subtypes which have been repeatedly described. Subdivision of performance into vectors composed of more than one dimension may reveal subtypes of cognitive profiles that will correspond to subtypes of learning disabilities. Finally, the CLQ blurs the distinction between high and low performers, the latter may be the ones with the reported "perceptual" problems.

The virtues of characterizing reading disabled individuals (or anyone else for that matter) by a single profile measure is partly theoretical, partly empirical. In the first place, a number of the subjects in the disabled population had *normal* performance on tests of left hemisphere function and above normal performance on tests of right hemisphere function; yet they had difficulty in reading. The parsimonious explanation is that the *asymmetry* of function is more crucial to reading than the absolute abilities themselves. The paradox is best illustrated by the comment of one parent when presented with her son's results: "Do you mean that if my son weren't so smart [with his right hemisphere] he would be able to read?" Indeed it would be consistent with these data that if the ability on left hemisphere functions was to remain the same and ability on the "right" tests was reduced, he might well have been a better reader. One thing for sure, his near normal performance on left hemisphere tasks was not predictive of his reading ability.

These data suggest that for the overwhelming majority of individuals referred for learning problems--problems that are primary and not secondary to neurological, psychological, education, or social conditions--the "right hemisphere" cognitive profile prevails; subjects perform better on tests attributed to the right hemisphere than on tests attributed to the left.

Similar correlative results were seen in forty unselected elementary and middle school students where performance on the standardized CLB was compared to achievement[2]. In general, it was best to have a cognitive profile favoring functions of the left hemisphere especially for above average performers. *None* of the sixteen subjects who performed better on *left* hemisphere tests *and* better than average overall had percentiles lower than 50 in the California Achievement Test (Total Battery). There were only two out of seven (29%) who performed better on left hemisphere tests but had below average performance (on the CLB) who scored below the 50th percentile in the total CAT. This should be compared to two out of four (50%) who performed below the 50th percentile on the CAT who had preference for right hemisphere tests (and performed below average on the CLB). There was only one out of thirteen subjects performing below the 50th percentile on the CAT who had a right hemisphere preference and an overall above-average CLB performance.

In comparing the "right" profile group (better on tests of right hemisphere function) to the "left" profile group who both performed less than average on the CLB as a whole, we find that the right profile group was significantly worse than the left group (p<.05) by about twenty-five percentage points on the Spelling (75% vs. 51%) and Language Expression 60% vs. 36%) Achievement Tests. There were also trends for lowered scores in Reading Vocabulary and Total Battery. The same trends carried over to "right" and "left" groups with above average CLB performance but these differences did not reach significance.

The reverse phenomenon also existed. Children who performed lower than average on the CLB yet excelled in some achievement tests, often had the "left hemisphere" profile. One "left hemisphere" subject performed two standard deviations *below* average on the CLB, yet had an overall CAT percentile of 63 with a *99* on the spelling test. Another female subject who was a bit above average overall had a cognitive profile strongly in favor of the *left* hemisphere with an appropriate total CAT of 63. But she had a 95 in reading, and 88 in spelling. Her parents complained that she could not get into the honors group because her measured IQ was too low. It appears that her verbal, left hemisphere skills were exceptional but that spatial skills were poor. Clearly this child would not be lost in an honors course involving language skills.

EVIDENCE FOR UNDERLYING CAUSES OF READING DISABILITIES

It appears, therefore, that for most reading-disabled individuals, the right hemisphere cognitive profile is *necessary* for the learning deficit. Of course, not all individuals who perform relatively better on tests of right hemisphere function are reading-disabled, so the profile is not *sufficient*. Nevertheless, it is reasonable to hypothesize that individuals with a right hemisphere preference will be *ct risk* for reading and perhaps other learning disabilities. While performance on cognitive tests may improve throughout development, relative performance on tests of cognitive style remain much the same (Witkin, Goodenough, & Karp, 1967). Therefore we might further hypothesize that if a hemispheric preference can be determined at a pre-reading age, then one might focus attention upon those preferring the right hemisphere in order to enhance the chances of normal reading acquisition.

We have some preliminary cross-sectional data collected on about thirty children of the first three elementary grades in the public school[3]. About half the subjects were selected by their teachers because of "adjustment problems"; the other half were selected because they had no adjustment problems. The testers were "blind" as to the type of subject. Tests of the function of the right and left cerebral hemispheres were adapted from the Cognitive Laterality Battery and administered on an individual basis. For the right hemisphere, there was a test of form perception (closure), fitting of a puzzle piece which combines pattern perception and orientation, and point localization. For the left hemisphere, there were three tests of serial ordering using sounds, numbers, and visually-presented circles. The stimuli of each series were given in a specific sequence which the subject had to report in the correct serial order. The word production (fluency) test required the subject reciting as many words as possible in a given category.

Since no norms were available, Z-scores were calculated on the population itself. As before, assessments of right (A) and left (P) hemispheric function were determined by averaging the Z-scores for hemisphere-appropriate tests. The cognitive profile was defined by the Cognitive Laterality Quotient (CLQ) which was the difference between average right and left hemispheric performance: CLQ=A-P. A measure of overall performance (the Cognitive Performance Quotient, CPQ) was obtained from the sum of the 2 hemispheric measures: CPQ=A+P. Achievement was assessed by subtests of the California Achievement Tests.

The results indicated that the greatest handicap was a cognitive profile favoring right hemisphere tests (that is, a CLQ>0) and a performance profile, CPQ, below average (that is, a CPQ<0). Most subjects with this profile performed virtually all tests and the Total below average (Table 1). The best profile was one favoring left hemisphere tests (CLQ<0) and overall performance greater than average (CPQ>0). Most subjects with this profile performed all tests and the Total above average. The other performance/profile combinations produced results in-between (Table 1).

The Reading Vocabulary subtest was most affected by cognitive profile. A right hemisphere profile predicted poor performance, a left hemisphere profile predicted good performance regardless of overall ability (CPQ). The distribution of subjects (N=30) over the four possible combinations of right/left cognitive profile and

Table 1. Performance on achievement tests in relation to cognitive profile (CLQ) and cognitive performance (CPQ)

Achievement Tests	CLQ+		CLQ-	
	CPQ-	CPQ+	CPQ-	CPQ+
Vocabulary	↓	↓	↑	↑
Comprehension	=	↑	↓	↑
Arithmetic Concepts	↓	↑	↓	↑
Arithmetic Computation	↓	↑	↑	↑
Language	↓	↑	↓	↑
Total Battery	↓	=	=	↑

above/below average Vocabulary performance was probably not random (p=0.062, Fisher Exact Test). By contrast, arithmetic Concepts and Reading Comprehension seemed to be influenced by overall performance. Their distributions for above/below average CPQ and above/below average subtest performance was also not random (p=0.019 and 0.060 for Arithmetic Concepts and Reading Comprehension, respectively; Fisher Exact Test).

The results of this pilot study indicate the cognitive profile, in addition to overall performance, may be important in determining factors for school achievement. But these data are limited both in the size and composition of the subject pool. Standardization on a large data pool of young (age<8) subjects and validation are yet to be performed.

Dys. Fam. B-D.

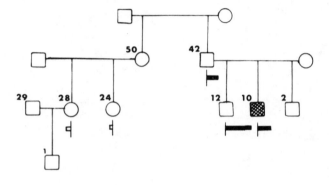

Dys. Fam. B-Sh.

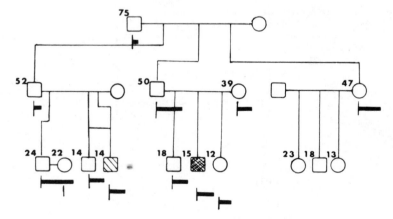

Fig. 2.   The CLQ for identified dyslexics and their family members.

The Genetic Aspects of Dyslexia

The genetic nature of dyslexia has long been recognized (Orton, 1943; Hallgren, 1950; Bakwin, 1973) although a model has never been determined. Suspecting that at least some specialized cognitive function is genetic (Bock & Kolakowski, 1973), we decided to observe the family patterns of cognitive asymmetry (Gordon, 1980). Accordingly, families in which there were identified dyslexic children were tested with the Cognitive Laterality Battery. The results were strikingly similar to those for the dyslexic children. There was a large, positive CLQ (but smaller than the dyslexics) in which tests of right hemisphere functions were performed better than tests of left hemisphere function. Furthermore, parents and siblings of both sexes had the same effects (Figure 2). For the most part, the families did not complain of reading difficulties.

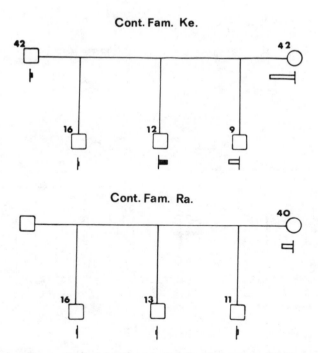

Fig. 3.   The CLQ for a "typical" family without reported dyslexic members.

Control families were chosen if they had no evidence of specific reading difficulties yet contained at least three male siblings (to assure our results were not due to the predominance of
males in the dyslexia population). The CLQ's were generally small
with no consistent direction (Figure 3). Thus it appears that
dyslexia occurs in a family with a history of right hemisphere
dominance even in the absence of familial learning problems. Perhaps genetic models have been using the wrong dependent variables.

Why does the asymmetrical ("right") hemisphere profile have
the potential for reading disabilities and why are family members
with a right hemisphere profile not exhibiting reading difficulties? Supplementary tests and analyses provide some insight. Two
reading exercises were administered to the dyslexic subjects and
the members of their families. In both tests, letters of three-
letter words were flashed on a screen one at a time but in their
correct spatial array (Figure 4). The words were constructed such
that they could be read in one of two ways: spatially and sequen-
tially. In the spatial version, the correct word was read according to the location of the letters, regardless of the order in
which they were flashed. ("CAT" in Figure 4). In the sequential
version, the correct word was read according to the sequence of
letters, regardless of their spatial location. ("ACT" in Figure
4).

The results showed that dyslexics were relatively better at
reading the words in the spatial version of the test while their
families preferred the sequential version. This interaction was
not likely to have occurred by chance ($F=3.47$, $p<0.05$). We may
speculate that dyslexics are using a qualitatively different reading strategy than their families. The dyslexic strategy appears
to be related to right hemisphere processing while the strategy of
the dyslexic's family is more related to left hemisphere function.
Are dyslexics "locked in" to the right hemisphere mode of processing whether or not it is the most efficient? Further analysis of
the data support this view.

It was found that the dyslexics had a significant correlation
between performance on the *spatial* reading test and measures of
both right hemisphere and left hemisphere function. The parents
of the dyslexics had none of these correlations. The siblings had
significant correlations between each of the reading tests and
tests associated with the right hemisphere but not the left. It
appears that the dyslexics have one cognitive processing mode
(resembling functions attributed to the right hemisphere) and it
is this mode that is used for all reading tasks as well as all
cognitive tasks. The family members, on the other hand, apparently are more flexible. They may use a mode that is more appropriate to the requirements of the task.

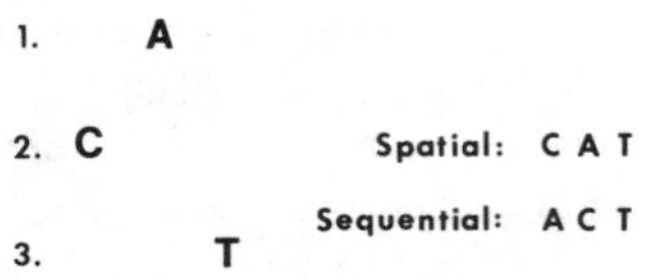

1.   **A**

2. **C**   Spatial: C A T

                           Sequential: A C T
3.   **T**

Fig. 4.   Reading test in which letters of 3-letter words are
           flashed sequentially. Responses may be according to
           either the *sequence* of letters or the spatial array.

        But *why* are dyslexics locked into this one mode of process-
ing? There is a pervading impression that lateral dominance, such
as handedness and eyedness, of dyslexics is weaker than in the
normal population. Although ear dominance is questionably affected (Gordon, 1980), a tendency toward bilaterality does appear to
exist for spatial functions (Witelson, 1977). We can speculate,
then, that genetic instructions have produced an anomaly in development whereby both cerebral hemispheres become organized in the
same way--that which resembles the organization of the right brain
alone. This is probably not an "all or none" phenomenon so that
different individuals have differing degrees of bilaterialization
of right hemisphericity. Functions normally attributed to the
left hemisphere may still exist unilaterally in that hemisphere,
thus explaining residual speech dominance. However, left hemisphere ability is reduced due to interference from right hemisphere mechanisms (Levy, 1976).

REMEDIATION

        Studies that evaluate remedial methods usually have built-in
biases, which are not adequately controlled in order to prove that
a particular method is more successful than its competitors. A
number of different methods exist, many of which describe
approaches, such as the Orton-Gillingham, or programs such as
PEECH (Karnes, 1980) or TEACH (Hagin, Silver, & Kreeger, 1976).
Often the evidence of success is only a comparison to
"conventional" intervention or to no intervention at all (Hagin,
Silver, & Beecher, 1978). Intervention programs are based on such
practical matters as student interest and material relevance to
more theoretical considerations such as acquisition of language.
Thus the "High Interest, Low Reading" series captures the unmoti-
vated, while another technique introduces grammatical elements of
language in a specified sequence at regular intervals in an effort
to slow down the learning process to the rate of slow learners or

developers. However, evaluations of these methods as the "best" should include a number of controls: 1) number and quality of teacher-pupil contacts (teachers are more motivated and may work with their students more often in the new intervention); 2) use of novel or interesting materials; and, 3) the differences among the subjects themselves and their interaction with their home or school environment.

Certainly ethical and other practical considerations limit full control of experimental manipulations, but the apparent fact is that studies are concerned with establishing the efficacy of a new technique for *itself* rather than attempting to evaluate the theoretical foundations on which it was based. It would seem that if a cognitive foundation could be established, efforts to match training programs to different cognitive profiles would optimize remedial techniques. Otherwise research efforts to assess ever-increasing numbers of teaching techniques will continue to flood the market without resolution. With regard to the neuropsychological observation that reading disabled children have a cognitive profile favoring functions attributed to the right cerebral hemisphere, one of two strategies would seem reasonable. Either try to match the remediation techniques to stimulate the deficient hemispheric functions or, alternatively, match the remediation technique to take advantage of the better-developed, more intact hemisphere function. Since some of the apparently successful techniques already in wide use are reflective of left or right hemisphere functions, it would not be a difficult hypothesis to test.

Our guess for the most efficacious method is one that requires exercise of the weaker left hemisphere. Using the whole-word method to exploit the superior right hemisphere processing would only serve to reinforce the cognitive asymmetry, as well as maintain the apparent "locking in" of that mode of thought. Our view is that fear of failure or hopelessness on the part of the student would be best managed on a *psychological* level rather than skirting it by changing the teaching method. One would not say to a would-be football player, "You're quick and fast enough but your arms are weak, so let's practice running". We feel the analogy holds for the functions attributed to the left and right side of the brain. But until the appropriately controlled studies are performed we shall expect to hear success stories of students using either the phonics method or the whole word method, among others, without resolving the issue. All methods work to some degree; some better than others. The most efficacious is yet to be demonstrated.

FOOTNOTES

1. These data were collected in collaboration with B.Z. Harness,
    M.D., and R. Epstein of the Department of Neurology, Rothchild
    University Hospital, Haifa, Israel.

2. Support by MH30915 to D. Kupfer. The cooperation of the
    Pittsburgh Public Schools is gratefully acknowledged.

3. Project supported by a grant to Western Psychiatric Institute
    and Clinic, University of Pittsburgh by the Richard King
    Mellon Foundation. Cooperation of the Pittsburgh Public
    Schools is gratefully acknowledged.

REFERENCES

Arnt, S. & Berger, D.E.   Cognitive mode and asymmetry in
    cerebral functioning. **Cortex**, 1978, 14, 78-86.
Badian, N.A. & Serwer, B.L. The identification of high risk
    children: A retrospective look at selection criteria.
    Journal of Learning Disabilities, 1975, 8, 283-287.
Bakker, D.J.   Temporal order, meaningfulness, and reading
    ability. **Perceptual and Motor Skills**, 1967, 24, 1027-
    1030.
Bakwin, H.   Reading disability in twins. **Developmental
    Medicine and Child Neurology**, 1973, 15, 184-187.
Bentin, S. & Gordon, H.W. Assessment of cognitive asymmetries
    in brain-damaged and normal subjects: Validation of a
    test battery. **Journal of Neurology, Neurosurgery, and
    Psychiatry**, 1979, 42, 715-723.
Benton, A. Developmental dyslexia. **Advances in Neurology
    V.7**, 1975, 1-47.
Benton, A.L., Levin, H.S., & Varney, N.R.   Tactile perception
    of direction in normal subjects. **Neurology**, 1973, 23,
    1248-1250.
Benton, A., Hannay, H.J., & Varney, N.R.   Visual perception of
    line direction in patients with unilateral brain disease.
    Neurology, 1975, 25, 907-910.
Bock, R.D. & Kolakowski, D.   Further evidence of sex-linked
    major-gene influence on human spatial visualizing abil-
    ity. **American Journal of Human Genetics**, 1973, 25, 1-14.
Boder, C. Developmental dyslexia: A diagnostic approach
    based on three atypical reading-spelling patterns. **Devel-
    opmental Medicine and Child Neurology**, 1973, 15, 663-687.
Bogen, J.E. & Gazzaniga, M.S. Cerebral commissurotomy in man:
    Minor hemisphere dominance for certain visuospatial func-
    tions. **Journal of Neurosurgery**, 1965, 23(4), 394-399.

Bogen, J.E., De Zure, R., Ten Houten, R.D., & Marsh, J.F. The other side of the brain IV: The A/P ratio. **Bulletin of the Los Angeles Neurological Societies**, 1972, 37, 49-61.

Bryden, M.P. Response bias and hemispheric differences in dot localization. **Perception and Psychophysics**, 1976, 19, 23-28.

Butters, N. & Barton, M. Effect of parietal lobe damage on the performance of reversible operations in space. **Neuropsychologia**, 1970, 8, 205-214.

Camp, B.W., Van Doornick, W.J., Frankenburg, W.K., & Lampe, J.M. Preschool developmental testing in prediction of school problems. **Clinical Pediatrics**, 1977, 16, 257-263.

Carmon, A. & Benton, A.L. Tactile perception of direction and number in patients with unilateral cerebral disease. **Neurology**, 1969, 19, 525-532.

Carmon, A. & Nachshon, I. Effect of unilateral brain damage on perception of temporal order. **Cortex**, 1971, 7, 410-418.

Cohen, G. Hemispheric differences in serial versus parallel processing. **Journal of Experimental Psychology**, 1973, 97, 349-356.

Combe, G. **A system of phrenology**. Edinburgh: MacLachlan, Stewart & Co., 1843.

De Renzi, E. & Scotti, G. The influence of spatial disorders in impairing tactual discrimination of shapes. **Cortex**, 1969, 5, 53-62.

De Renzi, E., Faglioni, P., & Scotti, G. Tactile spatial impairment and unilateral cerebral damage. **Journal of Nervous and Mental Disease**, 1968, 146, 468-475.

De Renzi, E., Faglioni, P., & Scotti, G. Judgment of spatial orientation in patients with focal brain damage. **Journal of Neurology, Neurosurgery, and Psychiatry**, 1971, 34, 489-495.

De Renzi, E., Faglioni, P., & Villa, P. Sequential memory for figures in brain-damaged patients. **Neuropsychologia**, 1977, 15, 43-49.

Doehring, D.G. & Hoshko, I.M. Classification of reading problems by the Q-technique of factor analysis. **Cortex**, 1977, 13, 281-294.

Efron, R. Temporal perception, aphasia, and deja vu. **Brain**, 1963, 86, 403-424.

Faglioni, P., Scotti, G., & Spinnler, H. The performance of brain-damaged patients in spatial localization of visual and tactile stimuli. **Brain**, 1971, 94, 443-454.

Farrar, J.E. & Leigh, J. Factors associated with reading failure. **Social Science and Medicine**, 1972, 6, 241-251.

Ferinden, W.E. & Jacobson, S. Early identification of learning disabilities. **Journal of Learning Disabilities**, 1970, 3, 589-593.

Fletcher, J.M. & Satz, P.   Developmental changes in neuro-psychological correlates of reading achievement: In six-year longitudinal follow-up. **Journal of Clinical Neuropsychology**, 1980, 2, 23-37.

Fountenot, D.J. & Benton, A.L. Tactile perception of direction in relation to hemispheric locus of brain. **Neuropsychologia**, 1971, **9**, 83-88.

Fountenot, D.J. & Benton, A.L. Perception of direction in the right and left visual fields. **Neuropsychologia**, 1972, **10**, 447-452.

Franco, L. & Sperry, R.W. Hemisphere lateralization for cognitive processing of geometry. **Neuropsychologia**, 1977, **15**, 107-114.

Furst, C.J. EEG alpha asymmetry and visuospatial performance. **Nature**, 1976, **260**, 254-255.

Geffen, G., Bradshaw, J.L., & Wallace, G. Interhemispheric effects on reaction time to verbal and nonverbal visual stimuli. **Journal of Experimental Psychology**, 1971, 87, 415-422.

Gordon, H.W.   Cognitive asymmetry in dyslexic families. **Neuropsychologia**, 1980, 18, 645-656.

Gordon, H.W. Left hemisphere dominance for rhythm elements in dichotically-presented melodies. **Cortex**, 1978, 14, 58-70.

Hagin, R.A., Silver, A.A., & Beecher, H. II TEACH: Learning tasks for the prevention of learning disabilities. **Journal of Learning Disabilities**, 1978, 11, 445-448.

Hagin, R.A., Silver, A.A., & Kreeger, H. **TEACH: Tasks for the prevention of learning disability.** New York:Walker Educational Book Corporation, 1976.

Hallgren, B. Specific dyslexia. **Acta Psychiatrica Neurologica Scandanavia (Supplement)**, 65, 1950.

Halperin, Y., Nachshon, I., & Carmon, A. Shift of ear superiority in dichotic listening to temporally patterned nonverbal stimuli. **Journal of the Acoustical Society of America**, 1973, 53, 46-50.

Haring, H.G. & Ridgway, R.W. Early identification of children with learning disabilities. **Exceptional Children**, 1967, **33**, 387-395.

Horan, M., Ashton, R., & Minto, J. Using ECT to study hemispheric specialization for sequential processes. **British Journal of Psychiatry**, 1980, 137, 119-115.

Husak, W.S. & Magill, R.A. Correlations among perceptual-motor ability, self-concept and reading achievement in early elementary grades. **Perceptual and Motor Skills**, 1979, **48**, 447-450.

Jackson, J.H.: (1874), **Medical press and circular**, 1:19 (reprinted in **Brain**, 1915, **38**, 80-103.)

Karnes, M.B. Cognitive/psycholinguistic model for educating young handicapped children. In W.M. Cruickshank (Ed.), **Approaches to learning**. Syracuse: Syracuse University Press, 1980.

Kaufman, A.F. Cerebral specialization and intelligence testing. **Journal of Research and Development in Education**, 1979, **12**, 96–107.

Kim, Y., Royer, F., Bonstelle, C., & Boller, F. Temporal sequencing of verbal and non-verbal materials: The effect of laterality of lesion. **Cortex**, 1980, **16**, 135–143.

Kimura, D. Spatial localization in left and right visual fields. **Canadian Journal of Psychology**, 1969, **23**, 445–458.

Levy, J. Cerebral lateralization and spatial ability. **Behavioral Genetics**, 1976, **6**, 171–188.

Levy, J. & Reid, M. Variations in writing posture and cerebral organization. **Science**, 1976, **194**, 337–339.

Levy, J., Trevarthen, C.B., & Sperry, R.W. Perception of chimeric figures following hemisphere deconnexion. **Brain**, 1972, **95**, 61–78.

Liberman, I.Y., Shankweiler, D., Fischer, F.W., & Carter, B. Explicit syllable and phoneme segmentation in the young child. **Journal of Experimental Child Psychology**, 1974, **18**, 201–212.

Mattis, S., French, J.H., & Rapin, I. Dyslexia in children and young adults: Three independent neurological syndromes. **Developmental Medicine and Child Neurology**, 1975, **17**, 150–163.

Milner, B. & Taylor, L.B. Right hemisphere superiority in tactile pattern after cerebral commissurotomy. **Neuropsychologia**, 1972, 10, 1–15.

Naidoo, S. **Specific dyslexia**. New York: John Wiley & Sons, 1972.

Nebes, R.D. Superiority of the minor hemisphere in commissurotomized man for the perception of part-whole relations. **Cortex**, 1971, 7, 333–349.

Nebes, R.D. Dominance of the minor hemisphere in commissurotomized man on a test of figural unification. **Brain**, 1972, **95**, 633–638.

Ornstein, R., Johnstone, J., Herron, J., & Swencionis, C. Differential right hemisphere engagement in visuospatial tasks. **Neuropsychologia**, 1980, **18**, 49–64.

Orton, S.T. Visual functions in strephosymbolia. **Archives of Ophthalmology**, 1943, **30**, 707–717.

Parsons, O., Vega, A., & Burn, J. Different psychological effects of lateralized brain damage. **Journal of Consulting and Clinical Psychology**, 1968, **33**, 551–587.

Patterson, A. & Zangwill, O.L. Disorders of visual space perception associated with lesions of the right cerebral hemisphere. **Brain**, 1944, **67**, 331–358.

Piercy, M. & Smythe, V.O.G. Right hemisphere dominance for certain nonverbal intellectual skills. **Brain**, 1962, 85, 775-790.

Ratcliff, G. Spatial thought, mental rotations and the right cerebral hemisphere. **Neuropsychologia**, 1979, 17, 49-54.

Richman, L.C. & Lindgren, S.D. Patterns of intellectual ability in children with verbal deficits. **Journal of Abnormal Child Psychology**, 1980, 8, 65-81.

Rizzolatti, G., Umilta, C., & Berlucchi, G. Opposite superiorities of the right and left cerebral hemispheres in discriminative reaction time to physiognomical and alphabetical material. **Brain**, 1971, 94, 431-442.

Rourke, B.P. & Orr, R.R. Prediction of the reading and spelling performance of normal and retarded readers: A four-year follow-up. **Journal of Abnormal Child Psychology**, 1977, 5, 9-20.

Rugel, R.P. WISC Subtest scores of disabled readers: A review with respect to Bannatyne's recategorization. **Journal of Learning Disabilities**, 1974, 7, 48-65.

Satz, P. & Sparrow, S. Specific developmental dyslexia: A theoretical formulation. In D. Bakker & P. Satz (Eds.), **Special reading disability**. Rotterdam, Rotterdam University Press: 1970.

Satz, P., Taylor, H.G., Friel, J., & Fletcher, J.M. Some developmental and predictive precursors of reading disabilities: A six year follow-up. In A.L. Benton & D. Pearl (Eds.), **Dyslexia: An appraisal of current knowledge**. New York: Oxford University Press, 1978.

Serwer, B.J., Shapiro, B.J., & Shapiro, P.P. Achievement prediction of "high risk" children, **Perceptual and Motor Skills**, 1972, 35, 347-354.

Smith, M.D., Coleman, J.M., Dokecki, P.R., & Davis, E.E. Recategorized WISC-R scores of learning disabled children, **Journal of Learning Disabilities**, 1977, 10, 437-443.

Tallal, P. & Piercy, M. Defects of nonverbal auditory perception in children with developmental aphasia. **Nature**, 1973, 241, 468-469.

Taylor, H.G., Satz, P., & Friel, J. Developmental dyslexia in relation to other childhood reading disorders: significance and clinical utility. **Reading Research Quarterly**, 1979, 15, 84-101.

Umilta, C., Bagnara, S., & Simion, F. Laterality effects for simple and complex geometric figures, and nonsense patterns. **Neuropsychologia**, 1978, 16, 43-49.

Umilta, C., Rizzolatti, G., Marzi, C.A., Zamboni, G., Franzini, C., Camardo, R., & Berlucchi, G. Hemispheric differences in the discrimition of line orientation. **Neuropsychologia**, 1974, 12, 165-174.

Vellutino, F.R. Toward an understanding of dyslexia: Psych-
    ological factors in specific reading disability.   In A.L.
    Benton & D. Pearl (Eds.), **Dyslexia: An appraisal of cur-
    rent knowledge.** New York: Oxford University Press, 1978.
Warrington, E.K. & Rabin, P. Perceptual matching in patients
    with cerebral lesions. **Neuropsychologia**, 1970, 8, 475–
    487.
Witelson, S.F. Hemispheric specialization for linquistic and
    nonlinquistic tactual perception using a dichotomous stim-
    ulation technique. **Cortex**, 1974, 10, 3–17.
Witelson, S.F. Developmental dyslexia: Two right hemispheres
    and none left. **Science**, 1977, 195, 309–311.
Witkin, H.A., Goodenough, D.R., & Karp, S.A. Stability of
    cognitive style from childhood to young adulthood. **Journal
    of Personality and Social Psychology**, 1967, 7, 291–300.
Zaidel, D. & Sperry, R.W. Performance on the Raven's Colored
    Progressive Matrices test by subjects with cerebral com-
    missurotomy. **Cortex**, 1973, 9, 34–39.
Zaidel, E. Lexical organization in the right hemisphere.   In
    P. Buser & A. Rougeul-Buser (Eds.), **Cerebral correlates of
    conscious experience INSERM symposium No. 6.** Amsterdam:
    Elsevier/North Holland Biomedical Press, 1978.
Zangwill, O.L.   **Cerebral dominance and its relations to
    psychological function.** Felinburgh: Oliver & Boyd, 1960.

MINIMAL BRAIN DYSFUNCTION IN PERSPECTIVE

H. Gerry Taylor

Children's Hospital of Pittsburgh
University of Pittsburgh School of Medicine
Pittsburgh, Pennsylvania

Although the term minimal brain dysfunction (MBD) recently has been supplanted by alternative nomenclature (DSM III, Spitzer, 1980), it continues to be applied in substance, if not in name. In part, this may reflect its relevance to a variety of problems (Birch, 1964; Denckla, 1977b; Touwen, 1978; Yule, 1978). Included within the rubric of MBD is a wide array of childhood disabilities, such as the failure to develop age-appropriate academic skills; attention deficits and hyperactivity; perceptual-motor, language, memory and cognitive deficiencies; difficulties in social adjustment; and, neurologic signs of EEG abnormalities (Conners, 1967; Clements, 1966; Gross & Wilson, 1974; Ochroch, 1981; Touwen & Prechtl, 1970; Wender, 1971). The incidence of these disorders varies markedly with estimates ranging as high as 50% for children seen at mental health centers, and between 5% to 20% for children in the school population (Becker, 1974; Minskoff, 1973; Schmitt, 1975; Wender, 1971).

In light of the diversity of problems to which the term MBD has been applied, a clear and unifying definition would seem essential. A study of the term's use in clinical practice fails, however, to reveal either clarity or consistency in its application. Multiple terms for MBD-type disorders are employed. Some labels stress abnormal brain status (e.g., brain-injured child, minimal brain damage), while other terms focus on certain behavioral disorders (e.g., dyslexia, hyperkinetic syndrome) (Clements & Peters, 1981). Formal definitions for MBD also vary tremendously. In some studies, MBD is defined on the basis of select behaviors, such as "soft" neurologic signs (Capute, Niedermeyer, & Richardson, 1968; Carey, McDevitt, & Baker, 1979; Peters & Spreen, 1979), or symptoms of hyperactivity (Satterfield, 1973; Stewart,

Thach, & Friedman, 1970). In other studies, a potpourri of symptoms is used to identify the disorder. In addition to hyperactivity and neurological soft signs, other criteria for definition may
include certain findings on psychometric testing, deficiencies
relative to expectations in academic skills, and abnormal EEGs
(Paine, Werry, & Quay, 1968).

One negative consequence of this state of affairs is the pro-
motion of interdisciplinary misunderstanding. The psychologist or
educator might want to defer the diagnosis of MBD to the physician, not realizing that the physician may base his judgment on
the psychologist's findings. Or the physician, perhaps discom-
forted by having to draw inferences about the brain based on
either his or a psychologist's examination, may begin referring
all children with MBD-like problems to a neurology service for a
CT scan or an EEG.

Such cross-disciplinary misunderstandings also promote misconceptions about the child. The educator may construe a diagnosis of MBD as indicative of a permanent defect about which nothing
can be done (Bateman, 1973), thereby presenting the physician with
a biased picture of the degree of the child's impairment. Another
unfortunate consequence that can occur is disciplinary isolation.
One discipline may see the other's involvement as unhelpful or
even obstructive. The definition of learning disability proposed
by Kirk in 1963 (cited in Kessler, 1980) and the parent/teacher
movement that followed, may have served as a primary catalyst for
positive changes in educational practices. However, it may also
have fostered greater professional isolation (Clements & Peters,
1973).

This chapter will begin by critically reviewing the historical and conceptual origins of MBD. Next, the utility and limitations of the concept of MBD will be discussed. Rather than summarize the substantial literature on this topic (de la Cruz, Fox,
& Roberts, 1973; Gardner, 1979; Ochroch, 1981; Rie, & Rie, 1980;
Rutter, 1982; Walzer, & Wolff, 1973; Wender, 1971), the effort
will be to clarify the MBD concept, trace its development, and
address its implications for research.

HISTORICAL ANTECEDENTS

Perhaps the most direct point of origin for the concept of
MBD was the recognition that brain damage can have distinct or
specific effects on behavior and cognition. Because certain behavior and learning disabilities were linked to specific brain
disorders, it seemed plausible to also implicate a neurologic abnormality for similar overt disorders, even when direct evidence
of CNS pathology was lacking.

Strauss and his associates (Strauss & Kephart, 1955; Strauss & Lehtinen, 1947; Strauss & Werner, 1942) are frequently identified with this line of reasoning. Their notion of "minimal brain injury" arose from the observation that there were distinct differences between mentally retarded children with and without a history of brain injury. Difficulties in abstract thinking, a tendency to persevere, impulsivity, inattentiveness, and perceptual disturbances appeared especially prominent in the exogenous brain-injured group. Although subsequent attempts to replicate their observations have often been unsuccessful (Baumeister & MacLean, 1979), the distinction between endogenous and exogenous retardation was adopted by numerous clinicians and researchers. The characteristics of brain injury in retardates were then generalized to brain-injured children of normal intelligence (Strauss & Lehtinen, 1947). So strong was their conviction that certain behaviors were specifically tied to brain damage that Strauss and Lehtinen (1947) extended the endogenous-exogenous concept even further by eliminating the requirement for a clearcut history of brain injury. Their justification for this was that the methods of ascertaining nervous system lesions were gross; consequently, they felt "justified in diagnosis on the basis of functional rather than neurological signs." While it was fallacious for Strauss and his associates to assume a one-to-one relationship between "functional" signs and brain status, their reasoning was in keeping with the thinking dominant at that time. According to such thinking, referred to by Ingalls and Gordon (1947) as the belief in the "biologic gradient of disease," brain damage could be expressed in varying degrees of severity, with the milder forms linked to less severe forms of developmental disability.

The historical roots of the MBD concept can, however, be traced to influences prior to the Straussian movement (Strother, 1973; Kessler, 1980). A number of predecessors had described the different types of aphasia and uniquely abnormal qualities of thinking and personality disturbance associated with various forms of brain disease in adults. Moreover, it was observed that certain types of brain pathology had specific effects on learning and behavior in children, without necessarily lowering other measures of developmental progress (Strauss & Kephart, 1955; Benton, 1962; Kessler, 1980). Case reports of language, attentional, and reading disorders in children for whom it was not possible to directly establish a neurologic disorder were also accumulating in the first half of this century. Nonetheless, their impairments were interpreted as further evidence for specific brain-behavior relationships. Descriptions of disorders such as congenital word-blindness (Hinshelwood, 1907), strephosymbolia (Orton, 1937), organic drivenness (Kahn & Cohen, 1934), and specific developmental dysphasia, dyslexia, and dysgraphia (Ingram, 1960) included speculations about their underlying brain pathology. Because of the diversity of these terms and their common adherence to brain-behavior models, they provided the essential stimulus to the formation of the broader, unifying concept of MBD as a neurological disorder.

Another stimulus for the MBD concept was the growing dissatisfaction with the prevailing psychosocial interpretation of many childhood disabilities (Clements & Peters, 1962). There was increasing awareness of the fact that many children who displayed learning problems appeared otherwise well-adjusted. It had also become clear that differences among children in learning and behavioral characteristics could not be sufficiently explained on the basis of the conditions under which they were reared. In this sense, MBD represented a backlash to an overextension of the psychogenic orientation (Gardner, 1979).

A final historical impetus for the MBD concept was the mounting indirect evidence for a biological-genetic basis for certain behavior and learning problems. This evidence, summarized by Clements and Peters (1962), consisted of reports that behavioral and learning disabilities were often familial and sex-related; documentation that the use of stimulant medications was an effective treatment; and, evidence for an association between these disabilities and complications of pregnancy and birth.

The hypothesis that brain disturbances could occur in subclinical forms, reflecting a gradient of severity, was receiving increasing empirical support in the period just prior to 1966. For example, Pasamanick and his associates (Kawi & Pasamanick, 1958; Pasamanick, Rogers, & Lilienfeld, 1956) demonstrated that there was a greater incidence of pre- and perinatal complications in children who were referred for behavioral and reading problems than in a nonreferred comparison group. These and other behavioral disturbances, which they described along a "continuum of reproductive casualty," were hypothesized to be due to brain damage which was too minor to produce more obvious neurological impairment, but which nonetheless resulted in "cerebral disorganization" (Knoblock & Pasamanick, 1959).

A DEFINITION

Because MBD is more fairly construed as a concept than as a specific diagnosis, the full meaning of the term cannot be ascertained by reference to a definition alone. Nevertheless, the definition proposed by Clements (1966) represents a culmination of the above noted historical trends, and is thus more than a definition in the usual sense of the word. Hence, a detailed examination of the definition advanced by Clements provides a means for further delineating the concept. Clements' definition summarized the views of an MBD Task Force on Terminology and Identification that was jointly sponsored by the National Society for Crippled

Children and Adults, and the National Institute of Health's Institute of Neurological Diseases and Blindness. Even today, it is
widely acknowledged as the most authoritative statement on the
topic (Conners, 1967; Becker, 1974; Baumeister & MacLean, 1979;
Rie, 1980; Black, 1981; Ochroch, 1981).

In his monograph, Clements (1966) noted the diversity of
labels for various childhood behavioral and learning disabilities. Common to many of these labels was the presumption of brain
abnormality in cases where such abnormality could not be proved.
To clarify this essential feature, and to draw some boundaries of
coverage, Clements proposed that the term MBD refer to:

> ... children of near average, average or
> above average general intelligence with
> certain learning or behavioral disabili-
> ties ranging from mild to severe, which
> are associated with deviations of function
> of the central nervous system. These de-
> viations may manifest themselves in vari-
> ous combinations of impairment in percep-
> tion, conceptualization, language, memory,
> in control of attention, impulse, or motor
> function.

To fully appreciate this definition, it is first necessary to
consider the rationale for including only children of at least
near average intelligence. Also essential is an understanding of
what was meant by "certain learning or behavioral disabilities,"
"deviations of function of the central nervous system," and "various combinations of impairment." Each of these components will be
taken up in turn.

NEAR AVERAGE, AVERAGE, OR ABOVE AVERAGE GENERAL INTELLIGENCE

Restricting the MBD category to children of at least near
normal intelligence drew attention to the population of children
whose problems did not fall within previously established classifications. By requiring at least near average intelligence, MBD
was distinguished from the more traditional neurological categories where intellectual impairments were commonly found (e.g.,
epilepsy, mental retardation, cerebral palsy, sensory defects,
aphasia). This contrast in intelligence was paralleled by others.
Thus, the motor incoordination exhibited by MBD children was compared to the movement disorders associated with cerebral palsy;
and their perceptual and language disturbances were contrasted
with deafness, blindness, and aphasia. The emphasis on "mild,
borderline, or subclinical abnormal manifestations of motor, sensory, or intellectual function..." was, in fact, one reason for
the adjective "minimal" in the term MBD.

CERTAIN LEARNING AND BEHAVIORAL DISABILITIES

An especially broad range of disabilities were included within the category MBD. Clements (1966) listed nearly 100 signs and symptoms. These were broken down into 15 "preliminary categories." The list ranged from symptoms as general as test performance indicators, disorders of thinking processes, and variations in personality, to more delimited features including impairments of perception and concept-formation, specific neurologic indicators, and disorders of speech and communication. Clements did not imply that children had to manifest all of these characteristics in order to qualify for the MBD category, nor did he infer that all characteristics were equally prevalent. Instead, he advocated consideration of a sufficiently wide range of disabilities so that various subcategories might become apparent. As a step in this direction, the following 10 symptoms were described as being the most frequent: hyperactivity, perceptual-motor impairments, emotional lability, general coordination deficits, disorders of attention, impulsivity, disorders of memory and thinking, specific learning disabilities, disorders of speech and hearing, and equivocal neurological signs and electroencephalographic irregularities. Generally recognized psychiatric disturbance (e.g., childhood autism, psychosis, conduct disorders) were not included under the rubric of MBD. Exclusion of these latter disturbances was apparently based on the fact that they already fell within a well-established classification of dysfunction.

DEVIATION OF FUNCTION OF THE CENTRAL NERVOUS SYSTEM

The requirement that the learning and behavioral disabilities be associated with "deviations of function of the central nervous system" is a critical component of the definition. The notion of CNS antecedents expanded the range of biological factors to encompass "genetic variations, biochemical irregularities, perinatal brain insults, or the results of illness sustained during the years critical to the normal development and maturation of the central nervous system." As clarified in a later paper (Clements & Peters, 1973), the mere failure for whatever reason (excluding obvious psychosocial influences or verified brain disorders) to meet age-dependent expectations in learning or behavior would qualify as an instance of MBD. In the final analysis, this represents an extension of the concept of individual differences (Clements et al., 1971). Viewing the CNS as a source of deviation rather than outright impairment may also have served to orient discussion toward predispositions to develop disabilities. The actual manifestations of these disabilities would then be dependent on environmental expectations and pressures (Clements et al., 1971; Wender, 1971). Use of the term "deviation of function" thus allowed the CNS to take on a broader role and to be a relevant concern even when demonstrable damage or disease was not present.

But to preserve the distinction between MBD and definitive neurologic impairment, this expanded role could not encompass cases of actual damage or disease to the CNS. According to Clements (1966), MBD was to be dissociated from disorders accompanied by "findings severe enough to warrant inclusion in an established category, e.g., cerebral palsy, mental subnormality, sensory defects." Review of Clements' monograph and subsequent accounts of the MBD concept (Wender, 1971; Peters, Davis, Goolsby, & Clements, 1973) suggests that a child with a definitive history of brain damage, regardless of the exact consequences, would also be excluded from the MBD category. Seen from this perspective, Clements established the MBD category as a niche for those disorders for which clear evidence of neurological abnormality was lacking, but for which the status of the CNS was presumed to be a relevant consideration. Wolff and Hurwitz (1973) encapsulated this point when they stated that MBD might be conceived of as "minimal brain damage syndrome without evidence of brain damage." Whereas their use of this phrase was intended as critical, appreciation of the MBD tradition is readily apparent. More recently, John (1977), Kessler (1980) and Black (1981) have reemphasized this same important facet of the MBD concept.

In this sense, the definition of MBD is somewhat of a paradox. On the one hand, it promotes presumptions about CNS abnormalities as determinants of certain learning and behavioral disorders; and on the other hand, the discovery of definitive CNS correlates for these disorders precludes the label of MBD. The only way to reconcile these two features is to view the MBD category as a nosological "holding tank." In essence, the concept of MBD represents a plea for consideration of constitutional factors where none as yet have been discovered. Rather than delimiting the role of environmental factors as antecedents to behavioral or learning problems, the concept calls for consideration of a broader set of determinants.

Acknowledgement that CNS factors might be important despite the absence of outright damage helps to account for the use of the adjective "minimal" in MBD, and the replacement of the noun "damage" used in previous discussions of MBD-type disorders (Strauss & Kephart, 1955) by "dysfunction." Thus, the adjective "minimal" can be viewed not only as an attempt to distinguish MBD-type disabilities from those associated with known neurological disorders, but also as a means of acknowledging the insufficiency of direct evidence for brain abnormality (Benton, 1973; Rie, 1980).

VARIOUS COMBINATIONS OF IMPAIRMENT

A final element in Clements' definition is the statement that MBD-type disabilities occur in combination. By 1966 it was becoming increasingly apparent that the various disabilities for which a constitutional basis was suspected -- disorders such as specific learning problems, hyperactivity, language deficits -- often occur together (Laufer & Kenhoff, 1957). It is now recognized that children with mixed deficits constitute the majority of children in the MBD category (Clements et al., 1971; Peters, Romine, & Dykman, 1975; Denckla, 1977a). The thought behind Clements' acknowledgment of this fact seems to have been twofold. First, by studying several facets of what were believed to be constitutionally related disabilities, it was hoped that certain clinically recognizable patterns or clusters of symptoms would begin to emerge (e.g., hypokinetic and hyperkinetic syndromes, primary reading retardation). Apparently this assumption was that these existing clusters might be further clarified or other clusters identified by virtue of a wider scope of inquiry. Second, it was hoped that this broader framework could encourage identification of individual needs, and thus result in more effective management and remediation. In a later publication, Clements and Peters (1973) emphasized the importance of multi-faceted educational programs that take into account individual learning needs and limitations. Seen from this perspective, the all-inclusive nature of Clements' list of identifying behaviors is more understandable.

SHORTCOMINGS

Having examined the meaning of the term MBD from both historical and conceptual perspectives, the strengths and weaknesses of the MBD tradition as a whole can now be more fairly evaluated. In this section, problems that have arisen because of terminological ambiguity will be taken up first, followed by an examination of some of the problems inherent in the MBD concept.

One major drawback of the MBD concept is that it is liable to misconceptions. The contention of this review is that, in a historical sense, the term was never intended to serve as a diagnosis. Neither was it intended to imply a unitary or homogenous disorder, nor to suggest that abnormal brain status be taken for granted. Nevertheless, it is easy to understand why so many persons, both professional and lay, tend to equate "MBD" with brain damage despite lengthy explanations regarding the subtle differences (Schmitt, 1975). One of the negative consequences of the tendency to mistakenly interpret MBD as a sign of definitive brain pathology is that it engenders a sense of helplessness among teachers and parents (Bateman, 1973). Another unfortunate consequence is the false belief that it takes all responsibility off of the child and parents and that it renders psychotherapy irrelevant (Rourke, 1975; Dubey, 1976). The choice of the words "minimal brain dysfunction" to label this tradition may well contribute to such misconceptions. As the term itself implies, there is minimal dysfunction of the brain rather than of behavior (Denckla, 1977b).

Had another term been chosen, some of the confusion surrounding the MBD concept may have never arisen. Because of the complexity of its referent, it is unlikely that any simple catchword or phrase would prove adequate, and a substitute term would also be subject to the same misapplication. A better alternative may have been to emphasize the reasons for *suspecting* constitutional influences.

The shortcomings are not, however, merely limited to terminological issues or to problems inherent to the use of MBD as a specific diagnosis (Rourke, 1975). There are a wide variety of more fundamental limitations with the concept of MBD as delineated in Clements' (1966) monograph. One major conceptual problem is a tendency to exaggerate and oversimplify the characteristics of "major" brain disorder for the purposes of contrasting these features with those thought to identify MBD. The generalized loss in IQ often seen in the context of definitive neurologic disease, for example, is contrasted with the "more specific and circumscribed perceptual, intellectual, and memory deficits, falling within the MBD category" (Clements, 1966). The fact is that even unquestionable brain injury sometimes fails to produce demonstrable behavioral impairment, or yields only limited deficits in the context of grossly normal IQ (Benton, 1973; Rutter, 1982). Clements (1966) was accurate when he stated that abnormal brain status can have varying effects on one or more areas of function, including motor, sensory, or intellectual systems. However, there is little basis for his premise that, so long as IQ is preserved, "mild, borderline, or subclinical" forms of these deficits clearly distinguish MBD from established neurologic disease.

Such fallacious reasoning is but one manifestation of the MBD tradition's reliance on brain-behavior isomorphisms in arguing for constitutional influences. The argument is that if clear-cut brain damage results in severe impairments (e.g., cerebral palsy, epilepsy, mental retardation) then less severe insults are responsible for more minor types of behavioral dysfunctions. This line of reasoning has substantial historical precedence (Strother, 1973), and is perhaps best represented in the previously cited notions of the "biologic gradient of disease" (Ingalls & Gordon, 1974), and the "continuum of reproductive casualty" (Knoblock & Pasamanick, 1959). These two concepts are important insofar as they bring attention to the possibility of undetectable constitutional determinants for certain behavioral or learning dysfunctions. However, they also propagate the fallacies that: a) the more serious or extensive the behavioral problem, the greater or more likely is the brain pathology; b) the behavioral dysfunctions should always be viewed as originating, at least primarily, in brain pathology; and, c) because we cannot yet identify the CNS pathology, it must therefore be of mild degree. None of these implications can be empirically supported. As alluded to in the preceding paragraph, there is no direct relationship between the degree of structural damage to the brain and severity of behavioral impairment (Touwen, 1978; Rutter, 1982). There is also no way to determine the extent to which MBD disorders reflect constitutional factors as opposed to social or emotional factors (Kessler, 1980; Rie, 1980). Finally, there is no sound basis for presuming that if indeed pathology is present in some cases, it is mild in nature (Benton, 1973).

Another major conceptual problem is the misleading requirement that children with MBD have "near average, average, or above average general intelligence" (Clements, 1966). This restriction to the normal IQ range seems to imply that retarded persons have established neurologic disease. Whereas it is true that mental deficiency carries the implication of abnormal brain status, pathological correlates of retardation have proved nearly as elusive as those of MBD disorders (Gordon, 1977; Baumeister, & MacLean, 1979). A further point is that the behavioral hallmarks of MBD are also associated with retardation, as well as with a variety of emotional disturbances (Haywood, 1967). Another negative consequence of the emphasis on at least near normal IQ is the implication that intelligence measures are free from the effects of the child's specific deficits. Clearly, this is not the case (Doehring, 1978). There is a pronounced tendency for children who fall into the MBD category to perform on IQ tests in a manner which, although broadly normal by definition, tends to be somewhat substandard (Belmont, 1980).

A final conceptual limitation arises from a zealousness to view any failure to achieve up to behavioral or learning expectations, if not accountable for by social-emotional factors, as sufficient evidence for a constitutional determinant. As a result of this willingness, the MBD concept has been justifiably criticized as being over-inclusive (Yule, 1978). According to Schmitt (1975), MBD has come to be used in reference to "any child who does not quite conform to society's stereotype of normal children." The MBD concept provides no guidelines as to how one might weigh the influences of psychosocial factors (Rie, 1980). It also fails to specify how severe a problem must be before invoking "special" constitutional influences (Boll & Barth, 1980). Consequently, diagnosis of MBD tends to be subjective and, until recently, there has been little appreciation for the contextual dependency of identifying behaviors (Kalverboer, 1976; Gardner, 1979; Rutter, 1982). Because the diagnosis of MBD is often based on the exclusion of factors known to contribute to the disability, rather than on the identification of established constitutional features, it is open to the many pitfalls of definition by exclusion (Rourke, 1975; Satz & Fletcher, 1980).

SUPPORTING EVIDENCE

Although considerable, the above problems do not render the MBD concept scientifically useless. Ultimately, the merit of the concept rests on the extent to which certain learning and behavioral problems can be ascribed to constitutional factors. The discovery of previously undetected neuropathological correlates for disorders once considered MBD-like would serve as one means of verification. The direct approach, however, has had limited results, and is unlikely to yield much information until more refined noninvasive techniques are developed for examining the brain structure and physiochemistry of children (Rapin, 1981).

The validity of the concept appears then to rest primarily on the credibility of indirect or presumptive evidence for constitutional influences. Several recent reviews (Benton, 1975; Dubey, 1976; Schierberl, 1979; Rie, 1980; MacMahon, 1981; Rapoport & Ferguson, 1981; Rutter, 1982; Taylor & Fletcher, in press) have addressed the question of the biological validity of MBD. Despite a number of serious methodological limitations, there is substantial evidence that at least partially supports the relevance of constitutional factors. The strongest evidence is offered by studies demonstrating sex and familial aggregation of these disorders, increased incidence of pre- and perinatal complications, chronic developmental delays, congenital physical stigmata, physical growth retardation, and abnormalities in what Benton (1973) termed "infrabehavioral" responses (e.g., anomalous electrophysiological patterns, soft neurological signs, neuropsychological deficits). Thus far, there are only hints as to whether these presumptive indices are predictive of treatment, prognosis, and clinical symptomatology (Rutter, 1982; Taylor & Fletcher, in press). Nonetheless, the ability of these indices to discriminate MBD children from normal children sustains the credibility of the presumption of a constitutional basis for MBD.

POSITIVE OUTGROWTHS

A further virtue of the MBD concept is that it is at least partially responsible for several important developments in the study and treatment of childhood disabilities. For example, it has drawn attention to the likelihood that certain disabilities reflect inherent (i.e., brain-related) differences among children. It has also encouraged the recognition of mixed forms of the various disabilities within the MBD classification (e.g., the learning disabled child with a concomitant attention deficit). The MBD concept has, moreover, served to widen our perspective on individual differences. The notions of "temperament" (Thomas, Chess, & Birch, 1968), "normal organicity" (Harrison & McDermott, 1972), "constitutional predispositions" (Kagan, 1966), "maturational lag" (Bender, 1957), and "neurological immaturity" (Schmitt, 1975) are contemporary examples of this broadened view.

Another positive outgrowth of the MBD tradition is the refinement of psychological constructs pertaining to attentional, perceptual-motor, linguistic, and conceptual abilities. Since deficits in basic psychological processes are hypothesized to be manifestations of MBD disorders (Taylor & Fletcher, in press), it is not surprising that the MBD tradition has fostered the exploration of psychological deficits. The products of this research have been substantial. For example, research on hyperactivity has revealed that a number of discrete deficits (e.g., inability to sustain attention, impulsivity, distractibility) comprise this disorder (Barkley, 1981). In addition, neuropsychological investigations of learning-disabled children have revealed a wide range of specific deficits in linguistic and perceptual processes (Boder, 1973; Benton, 1975; Mattis, French & Rapin, 1975; Denckla, 1977b; Doehring & Hoshko, 1977; Satz & Morris, 1980; Rourke & Strang, 1981). Inquiry into the cognitive and neuropsychological correlates of MBD disorders remains a viable means by which to develop more useful definitions of specific disabilities, provide for earlier recognition of problems, and design more effective treatment methods. Furthermore, the MBD tradition has served as a catalyst for the recent upsurge of interest in brain structure and neurophysiology. While this research, to date, has limited applicability to the general class of MBD disorders (Rapin, 1981), studies of differences in brain morphology, neurotransmitter by-products, and electrophysiological responses may provide promising leads.

CONCLUSION

Examination of the use and historical origins of MBD reveals that it is a generic concept rather than a specific diagnosis. This term encompasses a wide range of disabilities that are not readily explainable on the basis of observable brain damage, sensory defects, mental retardation, or psychosocial disturbances. Learning disabilities and hyperactivity provide the most common examples of these disorders. Their inclusion in the MBD category represents the presumption of constitutional (biological and genetic) influences where direct evidence of such is absent or inconclusive. Overall, this presumption would seem to be justifiable.

The term MBD and the concept behind it are problematic. Despite the difficulties, the MBD tradition has been a fruitful one. It has led to greater focus on individual differences among children. It has fostered the development of more precise behavioral concepts, many of which have proven helpful in clinical work. And it has encouraged continued search for more definitive CNS correlates.

Used as a diagnosis, the term MBD is open to serious criticism. It implies that constitutional influences are known, and it promotes a stereotypic view of these disorders, as well as those disorders which are associated with definitive brain injury (Birch, 1964; Yule, 1978). Because the label "MBD" is so often mistaken to be a diagnosis, it would seem wise to drop this term in favor of descriptions of individual differences that emphasize the reasons for suspecting that a given problem may be the result of constitutional influences.

Applied as a concept, the term MBD cannot be so easily dismissed. The presumption of constitutional influences for disorders included in the MBD category has some justification and has proven to have heuristic value. Furthermore, the perspective toward childhood disabilities represented by the concept of MBD has served some useful purposes. In this sense, there would seem to be little merit to claims that MBD is devoid of meaning.

It is important to recognize, however, that the concept does have some serious limitations. Appreciation of these shortcomings is critical if the central tenet of the MBD concepts -- namely, the presumption of a constitutional basis -- is to remain a viable stimulus to research. One drawback is the false assumption that disabilities in the MBD group are distinct from those associated with brain injury, mental retardation, and emotional disturbance. There is, in fact, a good deal of overlap between these categories of childhood disability. Brain-injured children exhibit specific deficits (e.g., in reading or perceptual-motor function) that are similar to what is seen in children who have a learning disability or who exhibit hyperactivity without evidence of a brain injury (Benton, 1962). In addition, although retarded children are cognitively impaired, they nonetheless demonstrate differential patterns of neuropsychological impairment (Benton, 1970). There is also good reason for considering constitutional factors as contributors to adjustment and emotional problems (Rapoport & Ferguson, 1979). Problems in adjustment are in fact highly associated with certain MBD disorders, such as hyperactivity; and at least for some children, these disorders may be early manifestations of later psychiatric disturbance (Shaffer, 1978).

Comparisons between children with MBD disorders and those with other disabilities are, therefore, to be encouraged. Knowledge as to how definitive brain disease affects performance would suggest one means by which to further test the presumption of constitutional antecedents in cases where recognizable pathology is absent (Benton, 1974; Reitan, 1974). Comparisons of problem children with and without actual brain disease may also reveal important differences, underscoring the complexities of the brain-behavior relationships involved. The search for constitutional antecedents for various forms of mental retardation and psychiat-

ric disorder would likewise provide information as to the similarities and differences between these disorders and those within
the MBD category.

A second conceptual limitation stems from the dependence on
definition by exclusion (Rutter & Yule, 1975; Satz & Fletcher,
1980). One unfortunate consequence of such dependence is the absence of objective means by which to decide how serious a problem
must be to be included. Other undesirable consequences are that
it discourages the search for potential non-CNS factors that might
contribute to the problems, and that it fosters the belief that a
problem associated with known contributors (e.g., cultural deprivation, emotional disturbance) is necessarily distinct from a more
isolated problem (cf. Taylor, Satz, & Friel, 1979). Perhaps the
most serious limitation of definition by exclusion is that it
leads to sample heterogeneity. Although this limitation is best
illustrated by studies of children selected for "MBD," it also
defers meaningful research within such subcategories as learning
disability and hyperactivity. Even within these latter more
restricted domains, investigators have tended to group children
with diverse problems under a common label.

Recent trends in research show explicit recognition of these
limitations. In so doing, these trends have sustained the more
positive influences of the MBD tradition. Several contemporary
reviews (Benton, 1975, 1978; Yule, 1978; Rapoport & Ferguson,
1981; Rourke & Strang, 1981; Taylor, Fletcher, & Satz, 1982)
emphasize the need to group children on the basis of more specific
behavioral features. There are many instances in which this
approach already has paid off. As early as 1973, Conners demonstrated the possibility of isolating subgroups of MBD children
from a total MBD group and of discovering differential relationships between these clusterings and a variety of other variables
(e.g., response to medication, motor development, asymmetry of
cortical evoked responses). More recent examples from the literature on learning disabilities include the work of Mattis et al.
(1975), Satz and Morris (1980), and Rourke and Strang (1981).

A parallel trend is apparent in the research on hyperactivity. In a longitudinal investigation, Loney, Langhorne, and
Paternite (1978) found it useful to subgroup hyperactive children
according to the relative weighting of aggressive traits versus
more purely hyperactive behaviors. They discovered that the
children with aggressive features exhibited fewer soft neurological signs and came from families of lower socioeconomic status;
whereas the children with relatively more hyperactivity per se
responded better to stimulant medication and had more visual-motor
deficiencies. The two subgroups of hyperactive children were also
distinguished on the basis of their parental and peer relationships. A somewhat similar observation has been made by Stewart,

Cummings, Singer, and DeBlois (1981). They found that hyperactive children with a conduct disorder were more like children with a conduct disorder alone than they were like children with hyperactivity alone. The group of hyperactive-only children additionally had a higher incidence of learning problems than did the hyperactive-conduct disordered group. Behavioral analyses are further justified by evidence that the behaviors of children identified as hyperactive or as neurologically "non-optimal" are dependent on the context in which they are tested (Shaffer, McNamara, & Pincus, 1974; Kalverboer, 1976; Schierberl, 1979), and by indications that the situational pervasiveness of such problems may be an important variable (Rutter, 1982).

Constructing more useful definitions may demand that we become aware of the extent of normal variation in learning and behavioral patterns (Benton, 1974; Geschwind, 1974; Schmitt, 1975). As indicated earlier, one of the virtues of the MBD tradition is that it encompasses problems reflective of variations of normal behavior, or of failures to meet culturally related standards of performance. A study by Rutter and Yule (1975) demonstrates the value of incorporating developmental norms. These investigators found that specific reading retardation (defined as reading failure in excess of that predicted by regressing reading achievement on age and IQ) was more clearly related to a differential male:female ratio and slow reading process than was general reading retardation (defined as reading failure within expectations).

The final major shortcoming of the MBD concept is its tendency to be applied within a unitary causal framework. According to this model, MBD disorders are construed as direct reflections of constitutional factors rather than as products of both constitutional and nonconstitutional liabilities. Advocacy for a more interactional, multifactorial approach comes from numerous sources within the MBD literature (Touwen & Prechtl, 1970; Clements et al., 1971; Wender, 1971; Benton, 1973, 1978; Wolff & Hurwitz, 1973; Sameroff & Chandler, 1975; Doehring, 1978; Jansky, 1978; Baumeister & MacLean, 1979; Kenny, 1980; Rie, 1980). Birch (1964) captured the sentiment behind the interactional view in a statement that was made with reference to brain injury, but also applies equally well to MBD:

> We never see an individual whose disturbed behavior is a direct consequence of his brain damage. Instead, we see individuals with damage to the nervous system, which may have resulted in some primary disorganization, who have developed patterns of behavior in the course of atypical relations with the developmental environment,

including its interpersonal, objective,
and social features. The behavioral disturbances of children who come to our
notice are developmental products and not
merely manifestations of a damaged portion
of the brain.

The interactional view is also receiving mounting empirical
support. For example, Werner (1980) found that pre- and perinatal
complications bore a stronger relationship to developmental outcome in children from nonsupportive or stressful homes than for
those from more supportive and stimulating environments. Siegel
(1981) similarly observed that medical and developmental risk in
infancy was less likely to foreshadow later developmental delay in
children from relatively enriched home environments.

For the most part, however, the interactional approach rarely
has been applied. Fruitful extension of the MBD tradition may
require that we conceive of biological factors not as causal
agents, but as sources of "vulnerability" (Hertzig & Birch, 1968;
Rapoport & Ferguson, 1981). Following this approach, presumed
constitutional indices, such as early medical complications,
family history of disability, or neurodevelopmental deficiencies
would be regarded as predispositional factors. Whether these factors would lead to actual disability, and what form the disability
would take, would then depend on a variety of other variables. The
latter might include others' expectations of and reactions to the
child, the degree of social/cultural advantage available to the
child, and the child's level of social/emotional adjustment and
adaptability. Investigations of these factors would complement
research on children selected according to specific performance
criteria (Harrison & McDermott, 1972; Rapoport & Ferguson, 1981).
Both approaches are necessary if the MBD tradition is to be mean-
ingfully extended, and both will demand coordinated input from a
variety of disciplines. Abandoning the MBD label for less misleading terms, such as "attention deficit disorder" and "specific
developmental disorder" (DSM III) may aid in this process. Simply
dismissing the label, however, will not alone suffice to remind us
of the developmental and biological complexities of many forms of
childhood disability.

ACKNOWLEDGMENTS

The author wishes to thank Drs. Jack Fletcher and Craig Liden for
their constructive comments on the manuscript, and members of the
Child Development Unit at the Children's Hospital of Pittsburgh
for critical discussion and reflections on the topic.

REFERENCES

Barkley, R.A. **Hyperactive children: A handbook for diagnosis and treatment.** New York: Guilford Press, 1981.

Bateman, B. Educational implications of minimal brain dysfunction. **Annals of the New York Academy of Sciences,** 1973, 205, 245–250.

Baumeister, A. & MacLean, W. Brain damage and mental retardation. In N.R. Ellis (Ed.), **Handbook of mental deficiency. Psychological theory and research** (2nd Edition). Hillsdale, N.J.: Lawrence Erlbaum Associates, 1979.

Becker, R. Minimal cerebral (brain) dysfunction – a clinical fact or neurological fiction? The syndrome critically reexamined in light of some hard neurological evidence. **Israel Annals of Psychiatry and Related Disciplines,** 1974, 12, 87–106.

Bender, L. Specific reading disability as a maturational lag. **Bulletin of the Orton Society,** 1957, 7, 9–18.

Belmont, L. Epidemiology. In H.E. Rie & E.D. Rie (Eds.), **Handbook of minimal brain dysfunctions: A critical review.** New York: John Wiley & Sons, 1980.

Benton, A. Behavioral indices of brain injury in school children. **Child Development,** 1962, 33, 199–208.

Benton, A. Neuropsychological aspects of mental retardation. **The Journal of Special Education,** 1970, 4, 3–11.

Benton, A. Minimal brain dysfunction from the neuropsychological point of view. **Annals of the New York Academy of Sciences,** 1973, 205, 29–37.

Benton, A. Clinical neuropsychology of childhood: An overview. In R.M. Reitan & L.A. Davison (Eds.), **Clinical neuropsychology: Current status and applications.** New York: Wiley, 1974.

Benton, A. Developmental dyslexia: Neurological aspects. In W.J. Friedlander (Eds.), **Advances in neurology (Vol. 7).** New York: Raven, 1975.

Benton, A. Some conclusions about dyslexia. In A.L. Benton & D. Pearl (Eds.), **Dyslexia: An appraisal of current knowledge.** New York: Oxford University Press, 1978.

Birch, H. The problem of "brain damage" in children. In H.G. Birch (Ed.), **Brain damage in children: The biological and social aspects.** Baltimore: William & Wilkins, 1964.

Black, P. Epilogue: Brain dysfunction – toward a revised classification. In P. Black (Ed.), **Brain dysfunction children: Etiology, diagnosis, and management.** New York: Raven, 1981.

Boder, E. Development dyslexia: A diagnostic approach based on three atypical reading–spelling patterns. **Developmental Medicine and Child Neurology,** 1973, 15, 663–687.

Boll, T. & Barth, J. Neuropsychology of brain damage in children. In S.B. Filskov & T.J. Boll (Eds.), **Handbook of clinical neuropsychology.** New York: Wiley, 1981.

Capute, A., Niedermeyer, E., & Richardson, F. The electroen-
    cephalogram in children with minimal cerebral dysfunction.
    Pediatrics, 1968, **41**, 1104.
Carey, W., McDevitt, S., & Baker, D. Differentiating minimal
    brain dysfunction and temperament. **Development Medicine and
    Child Neurology**, 1979, 21, 765-772.
Clements, S. **Minimal brain dysfunction in children - terminology
    and identification**. NINDB Monograph No. 3 Washington, D.C.:
    U.S. Public Health Service, 1966.
Clements, S., Davis, J., Edgington, R., Goolsby, C., & Peters, J.
    Two cases of learning disabilities. In L. Tarnopol (Ed.),
    Learning disorders in children. Boston: Little, Brown, Com-
    pany, 1971.
Clements, S. & Peters, J. Minimal brain dysfunction in the school
    age child. **Archives of General Psychiatry**, 1962, 6, 185-197.
Clements, S. & Peters, J. Psychoeducational programming for
    children with minimal brain dysfunctions. **Annals of the New
    York Academy of Sciences**, 1973, 205, 46-51.
Clements, S. & Peters, J. Syndromes of minimal brain dysfunc-
    tion. In P. Black (Ed.), **Brain dysfunction in children:
    Etiology, diagnosis, and management**. New York: Raven, 1981.
Conners, C. The syndrome on minimal brain dysfunction: Psy-
    chological aspects. **Pediatric Clinics of North America**,
    1967, 14, 749-766.
Conners, C. Psychological assessment of children with minimal
    brain dysfunction. **Annals of the New York Academy of
    Sciences**, 1973, **205**, 283-302.
Cruz, de la, F., Fox, B., & Roberts, R. (Eds.) **Minimal brain dys-
    function**. Annals of the New York Academy of Sciences, 205,
    1973.
Denckla, M. Minimal brain dysfunction. In J.S. Chall & A.F.
    Mirsky (Eds.), **Education and the brain**. Chicago: University
    of Chicago Press, 1978.
Denckla, M. Minimal brain dysfunction and dyslexia: Beyond diag-
    nosis by exclusion. In M.E. Blaw, I. Rapin, & M. Kinsbourne
    (Eds.), **Topics in child neurology**. New York: Spectrum, 1977.
    (b)
Doehring, D. The tangled web of behavioral research on develop-
    mental dyslexia. In A.L. Benton & D. Pearl (Eds.), **Dys-
    lexia: An appraisal of current knowledge**. New York: Oxford
    University Press, 1978.
Doehring, D. & Hoshko, I. Classification of reading problems by
    the Q-technique of factor analysis. **Cortex**, 1977, 13, 218-
    294.
Dubey, D. Organic factors in hyperkinesis: A critical evalua-
    tion. **American Journal of Orthopsychiatry**, 1976, 46, 353-366.
Gardner, R. **The objective diagnosis of minimal brain dysfunction**.
    Cresskill, N.J.: Creative Therapies, 1979.

Geschwind, N.   Disorders of higher cortical function in children.
    In N. Geschwind (Ed.), **Selected papers on language and the
    brain.** Dordrecht, Holland: D. Reidel, 1974.
Gordon, J.   Neuropsychology and mental retardation.   In I. Bialer
    & M. Sternlicht (Eds.), **The psychology of mental retardation:
    Issues and approaches.** New York: Psychological Dimensions,
    1977.
Gross, M. & Wilson, W.   **Minimal brain dysfunction: A clinical
    study of incidence, diagnosis, and treatment in over 1,000
    children.** New York: Brunner/Mazel, 1974.
Harrison, S. & McDermott, J.   **Childhood psychopathology: An
    anthology of basic readings.**   New York: International Univer-
    sities Press, 1972.
Haywood, H.   Perceptual handicap: Fact or artifact?   **Child Study,**
    1967, **28,** 2–14.
Hertzig, M. & Birch, H.   Neurological organization in psychi-
    atrically disturbed adolescents: A comparative consideration
    of sex differences.   **Archives of General Psychiatry,** 1968,
    19, 528–538.
Hinshelwood, J.   Four cases of congenital word–blindness occuring
    in the same family.   **The British Medical Journal,** 1907, 2,
    1229–1232.
Ingalls, T. & Gordon, J.   Epidemologic implications of develop-
    mental arrest.   **American Journal of Medical Sciences,** 1947,
    241, 322–328.
Ingram, T.   Pediatric aspects of specific developmental dysphasia,
    dyslexia, and dysgraphia.   **Cerebral Palsy Bulletin,** 1960, 2,
    254–277.
Jansky, J.   A critical review of "Some developmental and predic-
    tive precursors of reading disabilities." In A.L. Benton & D.
    Pearl (Eds.), **Dyslexia: An appraisal of current knowledge.**
    New York: Oxford University Press, 1978.
John, E.   **Neurometrics: Clinical applications of quantitative
    electrophysiology.**   New York: Lawrence Erlbaum Associates,
    1977.
Kagan, J.   Developmental studies in reflection and analysis.   In
    A.H. Kidd & J.L. Rivoire (Eds.), **Perceptual development of
    children.** New York: International Universities Press, 1966.
Kahn, E. & Cohen, L.   Organic drivenness: A brain stem syndrome
    and experience.   **New England Journal of Medicine,** 1934, **210,**
    748–756.
Kalverboer, A.   Neurobehavioral relationships in young children:
    Some concluding remarks on concepts and methods.   In R.M.
    Knights & D.J. Bakker (Eds.), **The neuropsychology of learning
    disorders: Theoretical approaches.**   Baltimore: University
    Park Press, 1976.
Kawi, A. & Pasamanick, B.   Prenatal and paranatal factors in the
    development of childhood reading skills.   **Monographs of the
    Society for Research in Child Development,** 1959, 24, Serial
    No. 73.

Kenny, T. Hyperactivity. In H.E. Rie and E.D. Rie (Eds.), **Hand-book of minimal brain dysfunctions: A critical review.** New York: John Wiley & Sons, 1980.

Kessler, J. History of minimal brain dysfunctions. In H.E. Rie and E.D. Rie (Eds.), **Handbook of minimal brain dysfunctions: A critical review.** New York: John Wiley & Sons, 1980.

Knobloch, H. & Pasamanick, B. Syndrome of minimal cerebral damage in infancy. **Journal of the American Medical Association,** 1959, **170,** 1384.

Laufer, M. & Denhoff, E. Hyperkinetic behavior syndrome in children. **Journal of Pediatrics,** 1957, **50,** 463–474.

Loney, J., Langhorne, J., & Paternite, C. An empirical basis for subgrouping the hyperactive/MBD syndrome. **Journal of Abnormal Psychology,** 1978, **87,** 431–441.

Mattis, S., French, J., & Rapin, I. Dyslexia in children and young adults: Three independent neuropsychological syndromes. **Developmental Medicine and Child Neurology,** 1975, **17,** 150–163.

McMahon, R. Biological factors in childhood hyperkinesis: A review of genetic and biochemical hypotheses. **Journal of Clinical Psychology,** 1981, **37,** 12–21.

Minskoff, G. Differential approaches to prevalence estimates of learning disabilities. **Annals of the New York Academy of Sciences,** 1973, **205,** 139–145.

Ochroch, R. A review of the minimal brain dysfunction syndrome. In R. Ochroch (Ed.), **The diagnosis and treatment of brain dysfunction in children: A clinical approach.** New York: Human Sciences Press, 1981.

Orton, S. **Reading, writing and speech problems in children.** New York: Norton, 1937.

Paine, R., Werry, J., & Quay, H. A study 'minimal cerebral dysfunction'. **Developmental Medicine and Child Neurology,** 1968, **10,** 505–520.

Pasamanick, B., Rogers, M., & Lilienfeld, A. Pregnancy experience and the development of childhood behavior disorder. **American Journal of Psychiatry,** 1956, **112,** 613.

Peter, N. & Spreen, O. Behavioral and personal adjustment of learning disabled children during adolescence and early adulthood: A follow-up study. **Journal of Clinical Neuropsychology,** 1979, **1,** 17–37.

Peters, J., Davis, J., Goolsby, C., & Clements, J. **Physicians handbook: Screening for MBD.** CIBA Medical Horizons, 1973.

Peters, J., Romine, J., & Dykman, R. A special neurological examination of children with learning disabilities. **Developmental Medicine and Child Neurology,** 1975, **17,** 63–78.

Rapin, I. Disorders of higher cerebral function in children: New investigative techniques. **Bulletin of the Orton Society,** 1981, **31,** 47–63.

Rapoport, J., & Ferguson, H. Biological validation of the hyper-kinetic syndrome. **Developmental Medicine and Child Neurology**, 1981, **23**, 667-682.

Reitan, R. Psychological effects of cerebral lesions in children of early school age. In R.M. Reitan & L.A. Davison (Eds.), **Clinical neuropsychology: Current status and applications.** New York: Wiley, 1974.

Rie, H. Definitional problems. In H.E. Rie & E.D. Rie (Eds.), **Handbook of minimal brain dysfunctions: A critical review.** New York: John Wiley & Sons, 1980.

Rie, H. & Rie, E. **Handbook of minimal brain dysfunctions: A critical review.** New York: John Wiley & Sons, 1980.

Rourke, B. Minimal brain dysfunction: Is diagnosis necessary? Paper presented at annual meeting of the American Psychological Association, Chicago, 1975.

Rourke, B. & Strang, J. Subtypes of reading and arithmetic abilities: A neuropsychological analysis. In M. Rutter (Ed.), **Behavioral syndromes of brain dysfunction in children.** New York: Guilford, 1981.

Rutter, M. Syndromes attributed to "minimal brain dysfunction" in childhood. **American Journal of Psychiatry**, 1982, **139**, 21-33.

Rutter, M. & Yule, W. The concept of specific reading retardation. **Journal of Child Psychology and Psychiatry**, 1975, **16**, 181-197.

Sameroff, A. & Chandler, M. Reproductive risk and the continuum of caretaking casualty. In F. Horowitz (Ed.), **Review of child development research (Vol. 4).** Chicago: University of Chicago Press, 1975.

Satterfield, J. EEG issues in children with minimal brain dysfunction. **Seminars in Psychiatry**, 1973, **5**, 35-46.

Satz, P. & Fletcher, J. Minimal brain dysfunctions: An appraisal of research concepts and methods. In H.E. Rie & E.D. Rie (Eds.), **Handbook of minimal brain dysfunctions: A critical review.** New York: John Wiley & Sons, 1980.

Satz, P. & Morris, R. Learning disability subtypes: A review. In F.J. Pirozzolo & M.C. Wittorck (Eds.), **Neuropsychological and cognitive processes in reading.** New York: Academic Press, 1981.

Schierberl, J. Physiological models of hyperactivity: An integrative review of the literature. **Journal of Clinical Child Psychology**, 1979, **8**, 163-172.

Schmitt, B. The minimal brain dysfunction myth. **American Journal of Diseases of Children**, 1975, **129**, 1313-1318.

Siegel, L. Infant tests as predictors of cognitive and language development at two years. **Child Development**, 1981, **52**, 545-557.

Shaffer, D., McNamara, M., & Pincus, J. Controlled observations on patterns of activity, attention, and impulsivity in brain-damaged and psychiatrically disturbed boys. **Psychological Medicine**, 1974, 4, 4-18.

Shaffer, D. "Soft" neurological signs and later psychiatric disorder -- a review. **Journal of Child Psychology and Psychiatry**, 1978, 19, 63-65.

Spitzer, R. **Diagnostic and statistical manual of mental disorder** (3rd edition). New York: American Psychiatric Association, 1980.

Stewart, M., Cummings, C., Singer, S., & DeBlois, C. The overlap between hyperactive and unsocialized aggressive children. **Journal of Child Psychology and Psychiatry**, 1981, 22, 35-45.

Stewart, M., Thach, B., & Freidin, M. Accidental posing and the hyperactive child syndrome. **Diseases of the Nervous System**, 1970, 31, 403, 407.

Strauss, A. & Kephart, N. **Psychopathology and education of the brain injured child** (Vol. 2.), New York: Grune & Stratton, 1955.

Strauss, A. & Lehtinen, L. **Psychopathology and education of the brain-injured child**. New York: Grune & Stratton, 1947.

Strauss, A. & Werner, H. Disorders of conceptual thinking in the brain-injured child. **Journal of Nervous and Mental Diseases**, 1942, 96, 153-172.

Strother, C. Minimal cerebral dysfunction: A historical overview. **Annals of the New York Academy of Sciences**, 1973, 205, 6-17.

Taylor, H., Fletcher, J., & Satz, P. Component processes in reading disabilities: Neuropsychological investigation of distinct reading subskill deficits. In R.N. Malatesha & P.G. Aaron (Eds.), **Reading disorders: Varieties and treatment**. New York: Academic Press, 1982.

Taylor, H. & Fletcher, J. Biological foundations of "special developmental disorders": Methods, findings, and future directions. **Journal of Clinical Child Psychiatry**, 1983, 12, 46-65.

Taylor, H., Satz, P., & Friel, J. Developmental dyslexia in relation to other childhood reading disorders: Significance and clinical utility. **Reading Research Quarterly**, 1979, 15, 84-101.

Thomas, A., Chess, S., & Birch, H. **Temperament and behavior disorders in children**. New York: New York University Park Press, 1968.

Touwen, B. Minimal brain dysfunction and minor neurological dysfunction. In A.F. Kalverboer, H.M. van Praag, & J. Mendlewicz (Eds.), **Advances in biological psychiatry (Vol. 1.), Minimal brain dysfunction: Fact or Fiction?** Basel: S. Karger, 1978.

Touwen, B. & Prechtl, H. **The neurological examination of the child with minor nervous dysfunction. Clinics in Developmental Medicine** (No. 38). Philadelphia: J.B. Lippincott, 1970.

Walzer, S. & Wolff, P. (Eds.), **Minimal cerebral dysfunction in children.** New York: Grune & Stratton, 1973.

Wender, P. **Minimal brain dysfunction in children.** New York: Wiley, 1971.

Werner, E. Environmental interaction in minimal brain dysfunctions. In H.E. Rie & E.D. Rie (Eds.), **Handbook of minimal brain dysfunctions: A critical review.** New York: John Wiley & Sons, 1980.

Werry, J. Organic factors in childhood psychopathology. In H.C. Quay & J.S. Werry (Eds.), **Psychopathological disorders of childhood.** New York: Wiley, 1972.

Wolff, P. & Hurwitz, I. Functional implications of the minimal brain damage syndrome. In S. Walzer & P.H. Wolff (Eds.), **Minimal cerebral dysfunction in children.** New York: Grune & Stratton, 1973.

Yule, W. Diagnosis: Developmental psychological assessment. In A. F. Kalverboer, H.M. van Praag & J. Mendlewicz (Eds.), **Advances in biological psychiatry (Vol. 1.), Minimal brain dysfunction: Fact or fiction?** Basel: S. Karger, 1978.

LIST OF CONTRIBUTORS

Kenneth M. Adams
Department of Psychiatry
Henry Ford Hospital
Detroit, Michigan

Verne S. Caviness, Jr.
Harvard Medical School
Southard Laboratory
Eunice Kennedy Shriver Center
Waltham, Massachusetts

Campbell Clark
Department of Nuclear Medicine
National Institute of Health
Bethesda, Maryland

David D. Crockett
Department of Psychiatry
Division of Psychology
University of British Columbia
Vancouver, British Columbia

Harold W. Gordon
Department of Psychiatry
University of Pittsburgh
School of Medicine
Pittsburgh, Pennsylvania

Lawrence Hartlage
Department of Neurology
Medical College of Georgia
Augusta, Georgia

Patricia L. Hartlage
Department of Neurology
Medical College of Georgia
Augusta, Georgia

Harry Klonoff
Department of Psychiatry
Division of Psychology
University of British Columbia
Vancouver, British Columbia

Nicolas S. Krawiecki
Department of Neurology
Medical College of Georgia
Augusta, Georgia

Byron P. Rourke
Department of Psychiatry
University of Windsor
Windsor, Ontario

Gregory T. Slomka
Department of Psychiatry
University of Pittsburgh
School of Medicine
Pittsburgh, Pennsylvania

Ralph E. Tarter
Department of Psychiatry
University of Pittsburgh
School of Medicine
Pittsburgh, Pennsylvania

H. Gerry Taylor
Children's Hospital of Pittsburgh
University of Pittsburgh
School of Medicine
Pittsburgh, Pennsylvania

Cathy Fultz Telzrow
Cuyahoga Special Education
Service Center
Cleveland, Ohio

Roger Williams
Harvard Medical School
Southard Laboratory
Eunice Kennedy Shriver Center
Waltham, Massachusetts